Feeling Fit

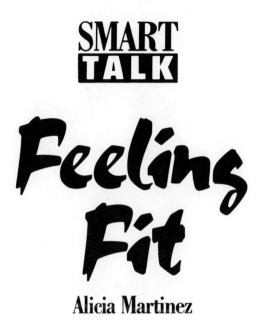

SMART
TALK

Feeling Fit

Alicia Martinez

Troll Associates

Library of Congress Cataloging-in-Publication Data

Martinez, Alicia.
    Feeling fit / by Alicia Martinez; illustrated by Donald Richey.
      p.   cm.—(Smart talk)
    Summary: Provides tips on exercising, nutrition, and self-esteem
for girls, ages ten to fourteen.
    ISBN 0-8167-2140-8 (lib. bdg.)   ISBN 0-8167-2141-6 (pbk.)
    1. Girls—Health and hygiene—Juvenile literature. 2. Physical
fitness—Juvenile literature. [1. Girls—Health and hygiene.
2. Physical fitness.] I. Richey, Donald, ill. II. Title.
III. Series.
    RA777.25.M37 1991
    613.7'043—dc20   90-10864

Table of Contents

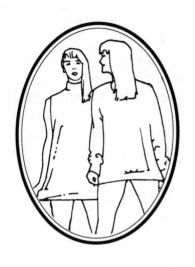

The Quest for the Perfect Body

The search for the perfect body obsesses many people. But we have a secret to tell you: You already have a great body. A "great body" is *your* body—as long as you like it and are proud of it, AND as long as you take care of it and keep it fit through good eating and exercise.

1

If there is a trick to having a great, fit body, it's simply finding the right balance: eating the right things, dressing in a flattering way and, of course, exercising. We're going to tell you how to achieve YOUR PERFECT BODY.

We'll discuss all sort of things about exercise and sports. But being fit also means eating right, understanding your body and, most importantly, liking yourself!

So, without further ado, pull on your sneakers, stretch out those muscles and let's get fit!

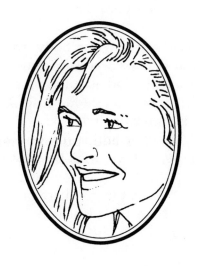

Feeling Good Is Looking Good

*I*magine that you only have one outfit in your entire wardrobe. That's it—nothing else to wear but that. And now imagine that this outfit is the only one you're ever going to have! You'd take care of it, wouldn't you?

That's the point. You only have one body, and you've got to keep it for the rest of your life. That's why taking care of your body—keeping it fit—is important.

Exercise makes both your body and your mind feel good. It also makes you *look* good. When you look good, you feel good about yourself—and when you feel good, you look good. And so it goes, on and on, in a wonderful circle.

There are a lot of scientific reasons why it's great to keep in shape, but we think that the way exercise makes you look and feel is the best reason of all. Feeling good and looking good are both very important, and exercise is the ideal way to achieve both goals.

NO BODY'S PERFECT

Although we're going to talk a lot about looking good—and about taking control and helping to shape your body—we want to stress one very important point: There is no such thing as The Perfect Body. There are only healthy bodies.

People used to get very hung up on body types—especially women's body types. If you look back over history, you'll see that society has almost always created ideals concerning women's bodies. Those ideals were arbitrary—some people decided that a specific body shape was desirable, and everyone else felt they had to conform. In the twenties, for example, the flapper look was in—very slim, small-breasted and boyish.

4

In the fifties, the voluptuous, curvy, Marilyn Monroe look was popular. All the movie idols had big busts and round hips, and the term "sweater girl" was coined for girls who wore tight sweaters to accentuate their bust lines.

Sometime in the late sixties, big bosoms lost their appeal, and being thin came back into vogue. Real thin. Wafer thin. And thin stayed in vogue through the seventies, but, by the eighties, wafer thin was out.

A couple of interesting things happened in the eighties. Women began to rebel against the unreasonable demands made on them in the name of fashion. After all, what if you just weren't born curvy or toothpick thin? Padded bras or starving were the only answers—and they weren't pleasant.

The fitness revolution also added something new—the idea that the ideal body is a body that's in the best shape it can be. This way of thinking gives *you* control over the way you look. You can determine the shape your body is in by exercising, eating well and taking care of yourself. Women and girls are no longer dependent on matching someone else's idea of what they should look like! More and more women are now realizing that they can be proud of their bodies—whatever type their body happens to be. The fact is that being attractive involves a lot more than just the externals. Beauty involves the internal stuff—how you feel, especially about yourself, and how you relate to other people.

FITNESS FACTS

Whenever you exert yourself physically, you'll notice that a couple of things start to happen: You huff and puff, and your heart starts pounding. This is exactly what *should* happen during exercise; it shows that you've taken the first step to becoming fit.

You've probably heard the terms "cardiovascular" and "aerobic" fairly often, but you may not be quite sure what they mean. *Cardiovascular* refers to the heart and the system of vessels that pump blood and carry oxygen throughout your system. *Aerobic* exercise improves your cardiovascular system by increasing both the amount of oxygen your lungs can process, and the efficiency with which your heart pumps the blood containing oxygen to all the cells of your body. This brings us back to the huffing and puffing and the pounding heart. The stronger you make your lungs and heart through aerobic exercise, the longer you can exert yourself without fatigue.

Think about it. Each time you exercise, you make your heart and lungs stronger—which, in turn, gives your body strength and greater energy. And that's the idea. But that isn't the only benefit of exercise. Besides increasing your heart and lung capacity, exercise also increases your stamina and strengthens your muscles. All this adds up to a healthier body—and a healthy body is a happy body.

THE BODY-MIND CONNECTION

Scientists have increasingly found that exercise has many beneficial effects on your emotions. First, there's the theory based on *endorphins*. These are hormones that appear to act as the body's own mood-lifters and painkillers. Endorphins are released into the blood stream during exercise. This accounts for the "high" that people feel when they're exercising, and why they feel so good for hours afterwards.

Another reason exercise makes you feel so good is that it allows you to release a lot of the tension and stress that normally gets bottled up. If you've ever wondered why jocks seem so calm and levelheaded, it's probably because they work off the stress during athletics, instead of getting angry at other people or at things they cannot control.

The final benefit of exercise is the least scientific, but it's still very real: Exercise increases your feelings of self-esteem, self-worth and self-confidence. No matter what kind of exercise you do, the benefits will begin to show. Your complexion will glow—because not only will your good health be reflected in your face, but also, people who are in good physical condition tend to have fewer skin problems. Your muscle tone will improve, and you will find that you begin to move with increased coordination and grace.

And when you look that good, you will inevitably begin to feel good, too. People will notice how good you look—and will mention it—and that attention is bound to increase your self-confidence level. An additional plus is that you burn calories faster because exercise also increases your metabolism. So the benefits will show in a slimmer, more toned body—which is always good for the ego!

POSITIVE ATTRACTION

It's not just your body that starts to look good. There's an intangible quality that comes with exercise—something you can't exactly see or touch. It's energy, and energy is attractive. If you think of your favorite performers—rock stars, actors, dancers—you'll realize that the one thing they all have in common is energy. Now think about people you've been around who have no energy—those dull people who don't want to do anything or go anywhere. You know how unattractive and boring that can be!

FITNESS NOW!

We realize that while you may believe everything that we just told you about the benefits of exercise, you may still wonder why you ought to begin an exercise program right now. After all, you're young. You probably think, as most people do, that *youth* and *fitness* automatically go together. Well, unfortunately, they don't. In order to be fit at any time of life, you have to work at it. But the good news is that this is the fitness generation. Never before have more people been into working out and being fit. Many of today's pop stars and film idols are in great shape, and the fit look is decidedly "in." So lace up those sneakers and join the fitness generation!

BEFORE YOU START

The following two Quick Checks will help determine how *you* measure up:

Quick Check #1: Breathing Test
To check your cardiovascular fitness, try running for five minutes at a comfortable pace. If you're out of breath before five minutes, or if you're very winded by the end, you may be out of shape.

Quick Check #2: Fit or Fat?
The percentage of fat vs. muscle in your body is very important. Some people may weigh more than others who are the same height, but they aren't overweight because their bodies are primarily made up of muscle. To check if you have excess fat, pinch the skin under your arm. If you can pinch more than an inch of skin and fat, you could probably stand to lose a few pounds.

Another way to determine your proper weight is to look in your mirror. This can tell you more about whether you're unfit or overweight than any scale can, but remember to be objective. Most girls tend to think that they are heavier than they are. So, if you think that you are a bit chunky, you're probably just fine. (The reason scales aren't very trustworthy is that weight is affected by things like bone structure, percentage of muscle as opposed to fat and even by your menstrual cycle—most girls will gain a few pounds around the time of their period.)

TAKING CHARGE
(OF YOUR CHANGING BODY)

Later on, we'll talk specifically about some of the changes that are taking place in your body. Generally, your muscles and bones are growing, and fat deposits are beginning to settle in different areas. All of these changes are a natural part of growing up, and will occur without your effort or help. But you do have some control over how your body takes shape. Muscle adds definition and form, which is why a firm, toned body looks so good. Using exercise, you can build some muscles, shape others and work to keep fat under control.

Anything you do now to strengthen your heart and lungs or increase your endurance and stamina will result in future benefits. The exercise patterns you establish today will be with you for the rest of your life. So, if you begin a regular routine of exercise and sports now, you'll find that it'll always come naturally to you. In fact, you'll even find that if you skip exercise for one reason or another you'll really miss it.

Do you want to lose weight? If you took the above test and decided that you are overweight, then exercise is the thing for you! Exercise curbs your appetite *and* burns calories. Some activities burn more calories than others and also speed up your metabolism (which means that you burn calories more quickly and gain weight less easily). The most effective exercises are the ones where you increase your heart rate and keep it at that pace for at least half an hour. In other words, aerobic activities such as running, cycling and even race walking will satisfy this requirement. A slow jog will help control your weight better than even the most energetic game of tennis, because in tennis you stop and start a lot. At this rhythm, your heart rate doesn't stay constant.

EXERCISE CALORIE COUNTER
(FOR ONE HOUR OF ACTIVITY)

Activity	Approximate Caloric Expenditure
Walking (2.5 mph)	145
Volleyball	170
Dancing (moderate)	175
Walking (4 mph)	265
Tennis	370
Cycling (10 mph)	420
Racquetball	450
Basketball	470
Dancing (vigorous)	570
Skiing (10 mph)	600
Running (9-minute mile)	650

Take Note: The more you weigh, the more calories you expend in an activity. But, of course, you may have to expend more to get to your weight goal.

EXERCISE IS SOCIAL!

Do you want to make friends? Fitness *does* lead to friendships. No matter what activity you choose, you'll find you'll meet people because those people who take up an activity love to talk about it. So, once you find other people doing what you're doing, it'll be easy to talk to them. Joining a team will give you more of an opportunity to see your new friends. And any type of group class—such as dance, aerobics or even swimming—could be a good place to meet people with similar interests. Working out, participating in sports and even walking around the block are great ways to make new friends—girls *and* boys!

I KNOW WHAT BOYS LIKE

We're about to tell you a very important secret about what boys like, and we hope you won't be too surprised. Boys like girls who like themselves. The most popular girls and women often aren't the ones who are the best-looking. But they are usually the ones who have the most confidence and self-assurance—the ones who like themselves.

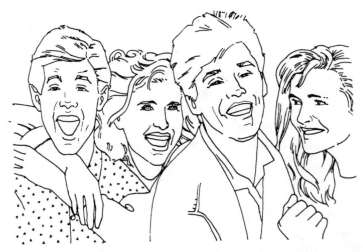

Exercise is a fabulous way to meet people and make new friends.

If you stop and think about it, this makes perfect sense. If you have self-confidence, you feel comfortable with yourself. And if you're self-assured, you make the people around you, even boys, feel at ease. That's because instead of being self-conscious—thinking things like "Does my hair look okay? . . . Gee, I hope he doesn't notice that pimple on my forehead . . . Oh, gosh, is my stomach sticking out?"—you can just relax and *be you*! You'll be fun to be with. And everyone, especially boys, likes being with people who are fun to be with!

Of course, liking yourself so that you can become self-confident doesn't always come naturally. For a lot of complicated reasons, some of us grow up feeling negative and critical about ourselves, especially about our looks. But the fact that it doesn't come naturally doesn't mean you can't achieve it with a little hard work. So try the following exercise to learn to like yourself and your body:

LIKING YOURSELF EXERCISE

Rules for this exercise: You must completely give up all negative thoughts and feelings about yourself and adopt only positive ones. Now, go through the following lists and write down those things you like about yourself and your body. You must choose at least three items on each list. (Hopefully, you will write down more!) Don't be overly modest or shy—no one will see your answers if you don't want them to.

MYSELF
I'm:

Smart
Funny
Cheerful
Friendly
Fun
A Good Friend
A Good Listener
Honest

Reliable
Helpful
Hard Working
Interested in Many Things
Interested in Ideas
Interested in People
Happy

MY BODY
I'm:

Tall
Short

Coordinated
Strong

I Have:

Nice Eyes
A Great Nose
A Nice Mouth
A Pretty Smile
Smooth Skin

Beautiful Hair
Nice Hands
Graceful Arms
Pretty Legs
A Well-proportioned Body

Once you've written them down, think about those good points. Repeat them to yourself. Congratulate yourself on them. After a while, we think you'll find more and more things to like about yourself. When you do, go back and add whatever applies to your list.

For all quizzes, please write your answers on a separate piece of paper.

☆☆   EXERCISE QUIZ   ☆☆

Answer true or false to the following ten questions:

1. *Exercise tires you out and makes you dull and boring.*
   True or False
2. *Exercise gives you strength, stamina and endurance.*
   True or False
3. *Aerobic exercise is exercise you perform in short bursts.*
   True or False
4. *You can get "high" from exercise.*
   True or False
5. *Exercise builds lean muscle and burns fat.*
   True or False.
6. *Exercise has no effect at all on your muscle tone—it just builds muscles.*
   True or False
7. *The more you exercise, the more you'll eat.*
   True or False
8. *You only burn calories when you are exercising.*
   True or False
9. *Working out can be a group exercise.*
   True or False
10. *Boys don't like girls who exercise.*
    True or False

Answers:

1. **False.** Exercise gives you energy, and energy is attractive. No one with energy could ever be considered dull and boring.

2. **True.** Exercise increases your heart and lung strength, thus increasing your strength, stamina and endurance.

3. **False.** Aerobic exercise is performed at a steady pace to keep your heart rate elevated.

4. **True.** Aerobic exercise releases endorphins, the body's own painkillers, and gives you a natural high.

5. **True.**

6. **False.** Exercise tones and shapes your muscles, but doesn't turn you into a body builder.

7. **False.** Exercise curbs your appetite.

8. **False.** Exercise makes you burn calories faster—but you burn calories all day, even when you're asleep.

9. **True.** You can exercise in any size group you want, and it's a fabulous way to meet people!

10. **False.** Boys like girls who feel good about themselves, and exercise is sure to make you feel good about yourself.

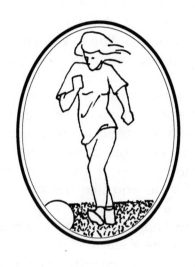

Finding Your Perfect Exercise

E xercise shouldn't be a chore—like cleaning your room or doing the dishes. Once you've started exercising seriously, participating in some sports activity or working out several times a week, you'll realize it's fun! But right now you're probably thinking: I know I need to get some exercise, but . . . It sounds boring, right? Wrong! The whole point is to find the type of exercise that will be fun. And if you give it a real chance, we'll guarantee you'll like it.

So, the goal of this chapter is to find something that you enjoy doing. The key is enjoyment. If you don't like what you're doing, you won't do it, and then you won't get healthier. So, let's consider for a moment what you would most *like* to do. Just think about which specific activity appeals to you. Which one makes you feel good when you visualize yourself doing it? Do you glow when you think of yourself running around a track or sprinting to a finish line? Or do you like the way you look in a bathing suit, gliding across a pool? Or do you picture yourself on a tennis court, serving, volleying and never missing a step?

Take this very unscientific factor into account when choosing your fitness activity. It is one of the most important factors, because what's vital is that you do *something*. If you don't like what you're doing, you simply won't do it. Think about it carefully, try lots of different things and don't limit yourself to just one sport or activity until you're really sure that *that's* what you want to do. The goal, after all, is to have fun!

☆☆ IMAGINATION QUIZ ☆☆

Are you really set to exercise? Take this quiz and find out!

1. *After school you like to:*
   a. Go over to a friend's house, share a gallon of ice cream and watch the soaps.

    b. Go home and read fitness books.

    c. Go for a quick, three-mile run and then do some *real* exercising.

2. *Looking at yourself, you see:*

    a. A future Olympic fan.

    b. A future Olympic reporter.

    c. A future Olympic diver.

3. *When someone throws a ball at you, you:*

    a. Duck for cover.

    b. Miss it and say, "But I thought Sally was going to get it."

    c. Catch it.

4. *Team sports make you think of:*

    a. Losing!

    b. Winning!

    c. Playing!

5. *You open your closet and see a pair of shorts and a pair of sneakers. You think to yourself:*

    a. Yuck! Those were in style *last* week.

    b. Wow, now all I need is a fabulous new top and I'm set!

    c. Wow! I have everything I need for aerobics!

If most of your answers are a's: Well, we're really glad you're reading this book. You need to change your outlook: Stop lounging around on the sidelines and *do* something.

If most of your answers are b's: Not bad. Your heart's probably in the right place even if your sneakers aren't. Now stop thinking about it and *do* it.

If most of your answers are c's: What can we say? You're the tops. Exercise your little heart out, but try not to overdo it. You could be forced to stop before you'd like to.

☆☆☆

WELL, WHAT I'M REALLY GOOD AT IS . . .

No matter how ready you are to exercise, you have to decide what you want to do before you begin. If you're not immediately drawn to one or more activities, then it's time to consider your aptitudes. The dictionary defines an aptitude as "an inclination, or tendency," or "a natural ability." And that's what we want you to explore—those natural abilities or inclinations you might have that would lead you to choose a particular exercise or sport. If you're finding it difficult to figure out what to try, there are several considerations which should come in handy. These are *body types, coordination* and *mind types.*

When pondering whether you have a body type or personality which would suggest pursuing one sport or another, there are some things to consider: Do you have an aptitude for any particular exercise?

Is there one for which your body type is particularly suited? Do your goals lead you to stress a certain area of development? Or do your circumstances limit your choices in any way? Let's take a look at each of these areas.

BODY TYPES, OR I'M TOO SHORT TO PLAY BASKETBALL!

Bodies come in thousands of different shapes and sizes—from short to tall, from petite to big-boned. And yes, certain bodies may be better suited to certain exercises and sports. That shouldn't surprise you if you stop and consider professional athletes, both male and female, and how the basic body sizes match up with certain sports. For example, gymnasts, runners and ballerinas tend to have petite body types; basketball players are tall and lean; and football players are big and broad. Think about what your body looks like. Do you look like a dancer or a basketball player or a sprinter? This might be a true indication of what you'd be good at.

Of course, there are exceptions to this rule, and we don't want you to think that you should avoid any exercise or sport just because your body type doesn't seem to be the perfect fit. There are short basketball players and big-boned ballerinas. You don't have to opt for the uneven bars instead of the b-ball court simply because you're 5'2". It's not just the body that matters, but how you use it. So, if you really like a sport, try it. You may even enjoy the challenge of overcoming the obstacle your body puts in your way.

COORDINATION, OR THE ABILITY TO MOVE TWO PARTS AT THE SAME TIME

Coordination may sound like a piece of cake to some of you, but to others it may be a very scary concept. Some people feel they just can't catch a ball or throw it straight or coordinate their feet to move at the same time that their arm is getting ready to swing!

If this sounds familiar, then we have some good news and some bad news. First the bad news: Most sports require some degree of coordination. If you choose a sport that involves hitting a ball, like tennis or volleyball, you're going to need eye-hand coordination. Even aerobics requires the ability to watch and listen to an instructor, and to move in response at the same time.

Now, for the good news: One of the best things you could possibly do to improve your coordination is—you guessed it—exercise. And you really will get better. Engaging in *any* fitness activity, regardless of the degree of coordination it requires, will improve your coordination simply because it will improve your control over your body. So, don't worry if you don't do everything perfectly at first. It may take some time, but we promise that before you know it, you won't even remember that you once worried about it at all.

MIND TYPES, OR I REALLY WANT TO WIN

In the same way certain body types are marginally more suited to one activity than another, your mental type might lead you to consider various options. If you would like to work on improving a mental attitude, such as confidence or discipline, there are activities which lend themselves to that as well.

For example, some activities require a great deal of *discipline*. If you're going to take up an individual sport—such as running or race walking—you're going to have to consistently get yourself out the door to do it. There'll probably be no class waiting for you, and no team expecting you to show up for practice. It's just you and your shoes. You've got to be the kind of girl who doesn't need to be told what to do—one who just does it. If you don't consider yourself disciplined, but would like to be, taking up a sport which requires discipline could be helpful.

Another mental attitude necessary for some activities is *concentration*. Some activities, particularly team and ball sports like tennis and volleyball, require you to really focus attention on the game— or you drop the ball. Activities that involve equipment, like cycling and skiing, also require intense concentration. Once again, those sports that require this attribute are also good for improving your concentration.

Competitiveness may also cause you to select one activity over another. If you're extremely competitive— that is, if you have a burning desire to win out over someone else at whatever you're doing—you'll probably be a great tennis player, and chances are the volleyball team would love to get their hands on you. Remember, if you often feel overwhelmed by competition, working on a competitive sport could help you learn ways of dealing with that feeling and taking charge yourself.

Discipline	Concentration	Competition
Walking	Dance	Team Sports
Running	Aerobics	Sports which
Swimming	Team Sports	have competi-
Cycling	Ball Sports	tions or meets—
Martial Arts	Cheerleading	such as
	Horseback Riding	swimming, golf,
	Ultimate Frisbee	horseback riding,
		gymnastics, etc.

REALITY CHECK

Practicalities. Yes, they are a bore, but they do matter. The most significant practicalities involved in choosing an exercise program are *cost* and the *availability of facilities*.

Some activities are fairly cheap and don't require much special training or special facilities. To *walk*, for example, you just need sneakers or walking shoes, shorts and a top. It's nice to have a park nearby; however, it's not essential, because with proper precautions you can walk safely along city streets.

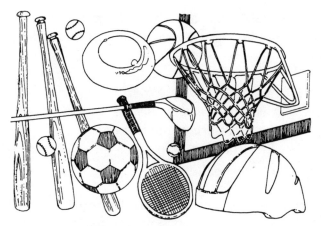

There are many different types of sports—find the one that's right for you!

Aerobics requires only sneakers or aerobic shoes and a leotard. But it does involve taking classes, or at least having a VCR and a tape so that you can work out at home.

Swimming can be very inexpensive if you have a pool or live near a lake, but the cost goes up if you have to join a club, which you'll almost certainly have to do in wintertime.

Cycling requires investment in a bicycle—plus maintenance—and a helmet.

Tennis requires some relatively inexpensive equipment—rackets and balls—plus the expense of a court (especially during the winter, when you'll probably have to play on an indoor court). But the real expense will be the lessons you'll need to start.

Skiing, both downhill and cross-country, requires travel (unless you live right near a resort), a lot of fairly expensive equipment, lift tickets, lessons, etc.

In general, here are the things to think about when considering the practicality of any exercise or sport:

- ✪ *Effectiveness in weight control.*
- ✪ *Probability of making friends.*
- ✪ *Cost of necessary equipment.*
- ✪ *Need for training.*
- ✪ *Need for special facilities.*

One thing to keep in mind, though, is that if you join a team, particularly a school team, they'll probably provide the equipment. If you're just starting an activity, and don't want to invest heavily until you're sure that you like it, try doing something at school—then get your own stuff once you're committed.

And it's not just the cost you must consider. Convenience is also an important factor. If it's very inconvenient for you to get to the pool, you're going to be less likely to go. Similarly, if tennis courts are hard to get to, you may *say* you're a tennis player, but talk doesn't keep you fit!

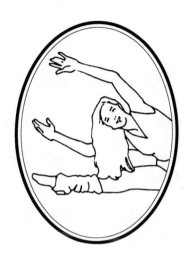

Let's Get Physical!

Wait! Stop! Hold everything. Before you even begin to exercise, there are some really important things you should learn. You need to know how to stretch, how to warm up, how to increase your exercise program in a healthful way and how to prevent one of the biggest obstacles in any fitness plan—boredom. These are The Rules of Success: If you get them down pat, then you'll be able to work out well, enjoy yourself and reduce the risk of an injury.

STRETCH FOR SUCCESS

No matter what exercise or sport you choose, it is absolutely vital that you warm up and stretch your muscles properly *before* you begin exercising. This is the key to feeling good and not getting hurt while you exercise.

Now, what we're about to tell you may sound a bit extreme, but we're going to say it anyway, because it's absolutely true:

Stretching is the most important part of exercise.

Stretching is the most important part of exercise.

Stretching is the most important part of exercise.

Why is stretching so important? Because the failure to warm up properly is one of the most frequent causes of sports injuries. When you're not using your muscles, they are "cold" and tight. When you use them, they get warm. The warmer muscles get, the smoother and more efficiently they work. If you try to force a cold muscle to do what a warm muscle could easily do, it just can't. It doesn't work as efficiently as it would if it were stretched. You could easily injure it; even if you don't, it will probably be stiff and painful from misuse the day after you exercise.

Stretching is a very natural activity. It loosens tight muscles and relieves tension. Just think about how you need to yawn and stretch when you wake up in the morning after not having moved your muscles much during the night. Stretching also begins the overall warm-up of your body by slowly raising your heart rate and drawing fluid to the joints so that you're less likely to get injured.

Now that we've convinced you to stretch *before* you exercise, we can tell you that it's equally important to stretch *after* you exercise. During exercise, you contract, or shorten, your muscles. And if you don't stretch them out again, they'll be very sore the next day.

SOME BASIC STRETCHES

Here are some basic stretches that will warm up your body and loosen your muscles. Try them out gently at first. If you experience any real pain, you're not doing it right—these stretches are not supposed to hurt. If you don't understand how to do them, or you continue to experience pain, ask your mom or dad or a gym teacher for help. They'll be glad to help, and will probably be able to explain it to you.

Before you begin, let's review the basic do's and don'ts of stretching.

DO's for Stretching

1. Start slowly and smoothly.
2. Remember to breathe deeply while you stretch.
3. Keep your stomach muscles contracted while you stretch.
4. Start by stretching large muscles, then move on to isolated, smaller muscles.
5. Hold each stretch for ten to fifteen seconds.

DON'Ts for Stretching

1. Never, never, never bounce.
2. Never, never, never swing.
3. Don't lock your joints when you stretch.
4. Don't overstretch—you'll know if you do because it will hurt.

★★★

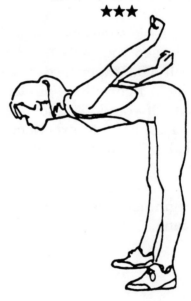

TOTAL BODY STRETCHES

Climbing: Stand with your legs six inches apart, arms extended straight up to the ceiling. Stretch your right arm up, and then your left, while you alternate moving up on your right and your left toes. Continue for twenty rounds.

Forward Bend: Stand with your legs about twelve inches apart and clasp your hands behind your back. Now bend slowly at the waist until your chest is parallel to the floor and your arms are raised in the air with your elbows extended. Hold for ten seconds. Repeat five times.

Crisscross: Starting from the last position, release your arms. Still bending at the waist, cross your right arm to your left toe, raise your left arm up toward the ceiling, and turn your head to look up to the ceiling, too. Hold for ten seconds, return to a standing position, and then do the same for the right side. Repeat twice on each side.

BACK STRETCHES

Knee Hug: Lie on your back with your knees bent (they should touch), feet flat on the floor. Bring both knees as close as you can to your chest without raising your hips from the floor. Wrapping your arms around your thighs (and under your knees), gently draw your knees a little closer to your chest. Hold for at least 20 seconds, and rest for 10 seconds. Repeat four times. (You can also alternate one knee, then the other. Hold and rest as above, and repeat twice for each leg.)

Knee Roll: Lie on your back with your knees together and bent, feet flat on the floor and your arms outstretched, palms down. Roll both knees over to one side until the outer knee touches the floor (or is as close as you can get it.) At this point, the top leg will be slightly higher than the bottom leg. Turn your head in the opposite direction while you do this. Hold the position for several seconds, then do the other side.

THIGH STRETCHES

Body Curl: Stand with your feet a few inches apart, stomach contracted, head up and knees slightly bent. Now, slowly begin to lower your head, curving your spine downward until your hands reach the floor. Then, slowly straighten your knees and feel the stretch in the back of your thighs. Repeat the entire process two or three times.

Thigh Stretch: Facing the wall or a chair, lean against it with your right hand, and with your left grasp the top of your right foot from behind. Then gently but firmly pull your heel toward your buttocks. Repeat twice on each leg.

LOWER LEG STRETCHES

Toe Touch: Stand up straight and swing your right foot over and across your left foot. Slowly bend from the waist, dropping your head and arms until your fingertips touch your toes. Repeat twice, alternating the leg that is in front.

Heel Touch: Stand in front of a wall, palms flat against the wall at about eye level. Push against the wall and take a step back onto the ball of your right foot. Now slowly extend your heel to the ground and feel the stretch. Hold this position for about ten to fifteen seconds. Repeat twice on each foot, alternating sides.

NECK AND ARM STRETCHES

Head Roll: You shouldn't actually *roll* your head during this exercise. Stand up straight with your arms at your sides and shoulders back. *Nod* your head forward, and then back up. Let it drop *gently* to the right and come back up, and then to the left gently and up. Finally, tilt your head back—not too far—then up. Repeat two or three times.

Shoulder Touch: Stand up straight with your feet comfortably apart. Hold your right arm out to the side, then reach behind your head and come as close as you can to touching your left shoulder blade. With your left arm, gently grab hold of your right elbow and gently push down on the elbow so you can touch your left shoulder blade with your right arm. Hold a few seconds, release and repeat on the other side.

WARMING UP

The basic aim of warming up is to gradually increase your heart rate. You see, it may be great for cars to be able to go from zero to sixty in thirty seconds, but it's awfully hard on your heart.

Your warm-up should include three to five minutes of aerobic activity done just a little more slowly than you do your main activity. For example, if you're going to run thirty minutes, you should start

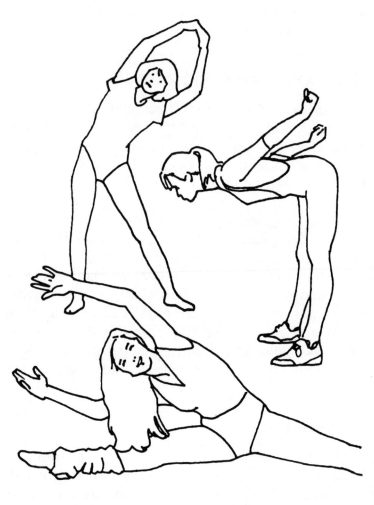

To avoid injuries, it is important to use correct form and stretch your muscles properly.

by walking briskly for three to five minutes. You can also do warm-ups as a part of your thirty-minute schedule.

COOLING DOWN

Cooling down is equally crucial. Think about that car coming to a screeching halt from sixty miles per hour; you could get awfully shaken up that way. So, at the end of your workout, take three to five minutes to gradually slow down from your maximum speed and intensity. Once again, you can include the cool-down in your thirty minutes or add it on. And, don't forget to stretch again after you've exercised!

NOT ALL EXERCISE IS ALIKE

Now that you've learned how to warm up and stretch out, it's time to find out how to form a total exercise plan. Keeping fit involves three different types of exercise: aerobic, anaerobic and conditioning.

Aerobic exercise, as we previously explained, really gets your heart and lungs going and keeps them working at a consistently high rate. Any activity that requires constant exertion and keeps your heart rate and breathing at a steady, elevated level—exercises such as jogging, swimming, jumping rope, etc.—is *aerobic* exercise.

Anaerobic exercises involve short, intense bursts of energy that leave you breathless for brief periods. Sprinting and the more intense ball sports, like racquetball and tennis, fall into this category.

Conditioning exercises require very little cardiovascular work, and concentrate mostly on stretching and strengthening muscles. Calisthenics, isometrics (exercise in which opposing muscles are contracted), and weightlifting all fall into this category.

All these types of exercise are great, but to get the most out of your exercise plan you should not rely exclusively on either anaerobic or conditioning exercises. In fact, the ideal formula is to take up one aerobic exercise and alternate it with an anaerobic or conditioning exercise. Let's look at how this works.

HOW MUCH? HOW OFTEN?

To get the real benefits of exercise—cardiovascular fitness, an increased metabolism, a sense of self-esteem and well-being: in short, the looking good and feeling good benefits—you really need to work at it, and *keep* working at it!

You should engage in an aerobic exercise for at least half an hour, three times a week. No kidding—that's the bare minimum. If that seems like a lot, remember it adds up to only an hour and a half a week. You spend upward of thirty hours a week in school getting your mind in shape. By comparison, an hour and a half to get your body in shape is a bargain!

If you let more than two days go by between sessions, you might begin to lose the benefits of exercising. So, you can't exercise on Friday, Saturday and Sunday and then let it go the rest of the week.

Of course, if you like, you can exercise even more

than that. You can increase the duration to one hour, three times a week, for example. Or you can increase the frequency to half an hour, six times a week. Or you can do both. But don't overdo, especially at the beginning. Overexertion is a sure way to get hurt and end your program before you've really had a chance to get started.

MAKING PROGRESS

Making progress in your exercise program—extending the amount of time spent and work done—should be a slow process. If you increase your exercise plan at a measured, steady rate, you'll be able to do it without undue injury, fatigue or frustration. A good rule of thumb is to increase your activity in increments of about ten percent a week. In other words, if you start by running one mile, don't increase to two miles the next week. Increase to a mile-and-a-bit. Then move up to a mile-and-a-quarter for the next week. This way, in a month or so, you'll be completely ready to move on to two miles.

At the beginning, start with just fifteen or twenty minutes of aerobic exercise per session, depending on how fit you are. If you're tuckered out after fifteen minutes, that's okay. Do fifteen minutes a day, three days a week, for one week. Then work up to seventeen minutes the next week, and then nineteen minutes the following week. Within a month and a half, you'll be doing the thirty minutes/three times a week plan with no problems. In the next chapter, we'll give you some sample progress schedules for several activities.

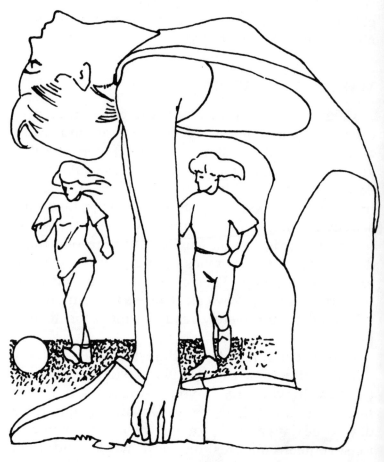

Cross-training and alternating activities are the best ways to guarantee a complete workout.

ALTERNATING ACTIVITIES AND
CROSS TRAINING

Since you'll be increasing the time and intensity of your aerobic exercise very slowly, it's a good idea to alternate with some anaerobic and conditioning exercises. For example, if you walk, run or cycle on Monday, Wednesday and Friday, you might want to take a yoga or calisthenics course on Saturdays. Or, you might play tennis or volleyball on Sunday.

You've probably heard people talking about cross training. This usually implies alternating two or more aerobic exercises, such as running and cycling, or swimming and skiing. There are a lot of benefits to both cross training and alternating activities.

If you do several aerobic activities, you double your aerobic time, plus, you also use different muscles in each activity and build all-around strength. For instance, jogging primarily develops the hamstrings (the back of your thighs), while cycling develops the quadriceps (the front of your thighs). Put the two together and your legs are going to look terrific!

Alternating an aerobic with a nonaerobic sport has benefits, too. Again, you increase your exercise time, you work different muscle groups and it's a great way to keep from getting bored.

Alternating indoor and outdoor exercises can also help you cope with severe weather conditions. You just may not want to run in a rain- or snowstorm, or when it's very humid. Try doing aerobics or indoor cycling on rainy days, and then go back outdoors when the weather is better.

Most importantly, cross training and alternating activities prevent boredom—so exercise stays fun!

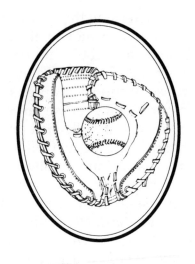

The Lowdown on Sports

*N*ow that you have all the basic information and you're psyched to get started, it's time for us to give you the whole scoop on the exercises and sports we keep mentioning. You'll need to know the basic movements and the benefits for each, as well as necessary equipment, safety tips and what to expect as a beginner.

JOGGING, RUNNING, WALKING AND RACE WALKING

These "locomotion" exercises are among the best for cardiovascular fitness, keeping your weight under control and toning your entire body. As you know, they require some discipline—you've got to get up and go at least three times a week. On the other hand, these are probably the easiest activities to try out—all you need is a good pair of sneakers (this is a good investment, since you can always use them for other sports and activities) and some comfortable clothes.

A MATTER OF SPEED AND BOUNCE

The differences between jogging/running and walking/race walking involve two elements: Speed is one, and bounce is the other. In terms of speed, walking speed is generally three to four miles per hour (about twenty minutes for one mile), while race walking speed should be six to eight miles per hour (or about ten minutes for one mile). The difference between running and jogging probably seems pretty obvious to you. Jogging is a slow, steady pace that can be sustained fairly easily over a number of miles (providing, of course, you're in good shape). Running is a considerably faster pace that is used for relatively short distances.

The bounce difference is somewhat more significant. In jogging and running, there is a point when both feet leave the ground; in walking and race walking, one foot is on the ground at all times.

41

Jogging and running, therefore, put a lot more stress on your body, because each time your foot strikes the ground it is coming down with your full weight behind it. (This stress is what causes the bounce when you come down.) So, although jogging and running are slightly better for burning calories and building muscles, walking and race walking are equally aerobic and much easier on your body.

POSTURE

The correct posture is important whether you try jogging or walking (or any other sport for that matter). You must stand up straight, head tall, shoulders back, stomach in. To see if your posture is correct at this very moment, take a sideways look at yourself in the mirror. If you slouch or your head is tilted forward and your spine is curved (standard poor posture), then you must learn to straighten up before you walk or run. Poor posture slows you down and forces you to use your muscles incorrectly, which guarantees aches the next day.

To improve your posture, just imagine that you're a puppet. You start out slightly crumpled. (Isn't that how you looked in the mirror?) Now a puppet master comes along and pulls your imaginary string, which extends through the top of your head down to the bottoms of your heels. As the puppet master pulls, you automatically re-align and straighten your body.

FORM

When you *walk*, swing your arms back and forth, moving each arm forward with the opposite foot. When you *jog* and *run*, on the other hand, you should hold your arms comfortably at your sides, keeping their movement to a minimum. *Race walking* requires that you move all of your body parts in very specific ways—and the movements don't come naturally. If you're interested in taking up this sport, you should purchase a book on the subject or get personalized instruction from a race walking club.

BEGINNER'S TIPS

In order to ease into your fitness program, it's probably a good idea to start with walking, and then move on to either race walking or jogging. Then, when you're feeling comfortable, you might want to pick up the pace and try running. Don't try to pick up the pace—graduate from walking to jogging, or from jogging to running—too quickly. Walk, jog or run at your normal pace; then, if you want, try a faster pace for five minutes and then return to your norm. This is called interval training, and it is a method employed by amateur and professional runners.

If you like the feeling you get from jogging and enjoy the sport, you can always develop a more serious regimen. Join a runner's club if there is one in your area, or get a book on running or race walking that goes into the specifics of form.

SAFETY TIPS

If you are walking or running on the sidewalk or road instead of a runner's track, watch out for uneven surfaces. Remember that the softer the surface, the less stress you put on your body. Good running shoes automatically protect you from all sorts of problems. (See Chapter Seven for more about sneakers.) Also, brightly colored clothing increases your visibility tremendously, which is especially useful if you're running at dusk or along a busy road. As for any outdoor sport, don't exercise outside if the temperature is below twenty degrees Fahrenheit or above ninety degrees Fahrenheit.

BEGINNER'S FOUR-WEEK PLAN
Walking / Jogging

Five minutes of stretching and warming up at the beginning, five minutes of stretching and cooling down at the end.

Week One: Three days a week. Fifteen minutes walking.

Week Two: Three days a week. Ten minutes walking, five minutes jogging.

Week Three: Three days a week. Ten minutes walking, ten minutes jogging.

Week Four: Four days a week. Twenty minutes, pick up pace in five minute intervals of walking/jogging or jogging/running as described above.

CYCLING AND SKATING

These activities are fun, aerobic—good for your cardiovascular system—and especially effective if you want to tone your lower body: They both give your legs a real workout. They're also great sports to alternate with running or walking because you use different leg muscles in these activities; if you alternate them, you're really giving your legs a full workout. Alternating cycling or skating with swimming also makes sense because then both your upper and your lower halves get lots of attention.

You do need equipment for both cycling and skating, but before you buy anything, try borrowing or renting supplies. And remember to keep your options open. You can cycle outdoors or indoors (with a stationary bike), and you can roller-skate outside or in an indoor rink. And don't forget about ice skating—it's a great winter sport and very social.

BEGINNER'S FOUR-WEEK PLAN
Skating

Five minutes of stretching and warming up at the beginning, five minutes of stretching and cooling down at the end.

Week One: Three days a week. Skate at a constant rate for twenty minutes.

Week Two: Three days a week. Skate at a constant rate for fifteen minutes, faster for five.

Week Three: Four days a week. Skate at a constant rate for fifteen minutes, faster for five.

Week Four: Four days a week. Skate at a constant rate for twenty minutes, faster for five.

BICYCLING FORM

There are three main points for proper bicycling form. Your saddle must be adjusted to the proper height, so that when your legs reach the bottom of the stroke they are still bent slightly at the knee. When you pedal, make sure you do so with a smooth, *circular* stroke. This means you really have to follow through at the bottom of the stroke. (Try imagining you are scraping mud off the bottom of your sneakers.) Your upper body and shoulders should be relaxed at all times, your elbows flexed yet relaxed, with a fairly firm handgrip.

BEGINNER'S FOUR-WEEK PLAN
Cycling (Outdoors)

Five minutes of stretching and warming up at the beginning, five minutes of stretching and cooling down at the end.

Weeks One and Two: Three days a week. Time remains constant at twenty minutes, three days a week. Increase mileage in small increments. Alternate hills with flat roads.

Week Three: Three days a week. Increase time to twenty-five minutes. Increase mileage in increments of two to three miles. Increase hills.

Week Four: Four days a week. Increase time, mileage and hills.

BEGINNER'S TIPS

You probably know the basics of both cycling and skating from trying them when you were a kid. Now you'll have to view them a little more seriously, since you'll be working at them at least three days a week for thirty minutes at a time (if you're not alternating them with another sport). As for equipment, it doesn't matter if your bike is a three-speed, a ten-speed or a mountain bike. They're all equally good for exercising.

You should start cycling at a slow yet steady pace, alternating between hills and level ground. As you improve, you can go a longer distance, as well as over more hilly terrain, at a faster pace. Remember, the faster the pace, the more muscle building you'll be doing.

BEGINNER'S FOUR-WEEK PLAN
Cycling (Indoors)

Five minutes of stretching and warming up at the beginning, five minutes of stretching and cooling down at the end.

Week One: Three days a week. Pedal ten minutes, rest two minutes, repeat.

Week Two: Three days a week. Pedal twelve minutes, rest two minutes, repeat.

Week Three: Four days a week. Pedal twelve minutes normal speed, pedal five minutes faster, rest two minutes, pedal ten minutes normal speed.

Week Four: Four days a week. Pedal ten minutes normal speed, pedal ten minutes faster, pedal ten minutes normal speed.

Remember to treat skating as an aerobic activity— keep at a steady pace! If you stop by the side of the rink to talk to your friends every time you go around, you won't be getting the full effect of the workout. Our advice is to skate consistently for thirty minutes and then stop to chat!

SAFETY TIPS

Skating and cycling can be a little riskier than walking or jogging, so you should take the proper precautions. If you're skating, get knee and elbow pads, and find a rink or nontraffic area. If you're cycling, make sure the bike is in good condition, wear bright clothes and reflectors if you have to ride in traffic (always ride with traffic, never against it) and don't even think about getting on a bike without wearing a helmet.

SWIMMING

Swimming is an all-around great sport, especially if there's a pool or a lake nearby! One of the reasons swimming is so good for you is that it puts very little stress on your body. The water cushions your body, and you're less likely to get stress-induced injuries. Although swimming also gives you an excellent overall workout—and is aerobic—it generally does more for your upper body strength than it does for your legs. You might choose to alternate swimming with a good lower body exercise like running or cycling. Swim once or twice a week and cycle or run two or three times a week.

BEGINNER'S TIPS

Although you probably already know how to swim, you might want to take a class—either at school, the local gym or a health club—so you can perfect your form. (Remember, classes are also great places to meet people!) Alternating strokes will help you develop different muscle groups. For example, you could alternate the crawl (which is particularly good for the legs) with the butterfly (which emphasizes your back and arms). If it's difficult for you to keep swimming for the allotted time in the beginning, try working with a kick board. You'll still be getting all the aerobic benefits of swimming, as well as a really good lower body workout, and you'll probably find it a lot easier.

BEGINNER'S FOUR-WEEK PLAN
Swimming

Five minutes of stretching and warming up at the beginning, five minutes of stretching and cooling down at the end.

Week One: Three days a week. Swim five minutes and rest two minutes, for a total of fifteen swimming minutes each day.

Week Two: Three days a week. Swim six minutes and rest two minutes, increase total swimming time to eighteen minutes.

Week Three: Four days a week. Swim ten minutes, rest two minutes, swim ten minutes.

Week Four: Four days a week. Swim eleven minutes, rest one minute. Repeat.

SAFETY TIPS

Lifeguards are there to keep you safe, not just to look good. So listen to them. If they say to stay out of the water, stay out! Never, never swim alone—a leg cramp in the deep end can be a very scary thing, unless there's a lifeguard there to help you!

AEROBICS, DANCE, GYMNASTICS AND CALISTHENICS

Not only do the activities in this group provide an excellent overall workout, but they are especially good if you want to work on specific parts of your body. They are also ideal if you want your workout to be social. You can, of course, do them at home with videotapes, but for a beginner it's best to learn the basic moves in a class.

Aerobics and dance classes combine a strenuous cardiovascular workout with firming exercises for specific parts of your body. Gymnastics and calisthenics don't have a cardiovascular effect because you can't keep up your heart rate for long periods of time while doing them. If you decide to take up these exercises, alternate them with aerobics, dance, running, cycling or swimming.

BEGINNER'S TIPS

All you need to get started are some good work-out shoes and an outfit that lets you really move. If you're shy or unsure, you can rent a videotape and see what it's all about before plunging into a class. Then, take a class at school or the local gym. Get a friend to go with you. But don't sign up for a year's membership until you're sure you like it.

If you decide to take classes, make sure they're for beginners. Don't be shy—let the instructor know that you're just starting. She or he will probably tell you to take it slowly at first and do only as much as you can. You'll also get that extra attention that could make things a lot easier. Gradually, you will be able to work up to more advanced classes and participate more often.

BEGINNER'S FOUR-WEEK PLAN
Overall Workout

Five minutes of stretching and warming up at the beginning, five minutes of stretching and cooling down at the end.

Week One: Three days a week. Twenty minutes a day.

Week Two: Three days a week. Twenty-three minutes a day.

Week Three: Four days a week. Twenty-five minutes a day.

Week Four: Four days a week. Thirty minutes a day.

SAFETY TIPS

Even though professional gymnasts make the sport look graceful and effortless, gymnastics can be difficult *and dangerous.* Never try gymnastics on your own. A qualified instructor should always be around to supervise.

TEAM AND PARTNER SPORTS

Ball sports are great for improving your concentration and eye–hand coordination. And if you like competition, then ball sports, such as tennis, racquetball, softball, volleyball, lacrosse, rugby, basketball or soccer, are for you! The same is true for hockey, rowing, competitive swimming and most other team sports. Some of these are more aerobic or anaerobic than others.

Aerobic	Aerobic/Anaerobic	Anaerobic
Rowing	Basketball	Tennis
Swimming	Soccer	Racquetball
	Rugby	Softball
	Hockey	Volleyball
	Lacrosse	

Of course, you will need a partner or a team for these sports. Check first at your school or in the community. Look into joining teams at school, and find out how you can sign up, or check out your local gym, girls' club or health club. Ask your friends if they're interested in any of these sports—it's always more fun to play sports with a buddy.

You might need some equipment, and that can be expensive. Start out by finding places—like your school—where you can borrow equipment, or at least rent it. Some tennis courts, for example, will rent you the rackets and balls.

We won't give you a schedule for these activities, because a lot depends on team schedules. But always remember: Don't overdo things at first, build up slowly, take all the safety precautions your instructor suggests and, most of all, have fun!

ADDITIONAL SPORTS AND ACTIVITIES

We obviously haven't listed every single sport above. There are many more that you can try. Here are some others that we find particularly fun and engaging:

- ✪ *Horseback Riding*
- ✪ *Skiing*
- ✪ *Water-skiing*
- ✪ *Martial Arts*
- ✪ *Cheerleading*
- ✪ *Ultimate Frisbee*
- ✪ *Skateboarding*
- ✪ *Jumping Rope or Double-Dutch*

- *Synchronized Swimming*
- *Track and Field*
- *Windsurfing*
- *And many, many more!!*

Go ahead and try a couple! You just might discover that you're an athlete at heart.

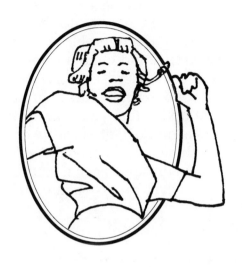

Gain without Pain

*B*y now you should have a better idea of the sports you're going to try. You're all ready to start. This is the fun part! Chances are you're going to love it; in fact, you might love it so much that you'll be tempted to overdo it. Or you just might want to jump right in without taking the time to stretch or warm up. You might even end up ignoring something that's hurting you and could hold you back. All these things could lead to trouble.

You have to know how to exercise properly, and how to take care of any problems that might arise. Take it easy at first and build up slowly. The fastest way to end your exercise program is to get too enthusiastic, overextend yourself or neglect a problem and end up hurting yourself.

There are a number of rules to remember, and we'll review them in this chapter. We'll also give you a brief lesson in first aid. Then if you become injured you'll know what to do—and you'll heal more quickly.

PREVENTION FIRST

Here are the most common reasons people get hurt:

- *They try to do too much, too soon.*
- *They don't stretch before and after exercise.*
- *They don't wear the right shoes and/or clothing.*
- *They don't drink enough water.*

We'll go over these one at a time, because they are extremely important and you should know what to do in order to have a healthy and enjoyable exercise experience.

THE TOO-MUCH-TOO-SOON SYNDROME

It's great to get excited about your exercise program! But in order to make real progress, you have to take it slowly. That's hard to do sometimes. There are days when you're feeling really good, and you just want to keep going. Like when you've just run three miles and you begin to feel that sense of elation—you're sure you can do two more, at least. Well, don't. Unless you work up to it slowly, you run the risk of hurting yourself. If that happens, you'll just end up slowing down your progress.

We explained in Chapter Three that you should increase your workouts in increments of about ten percent a week until you get comfortable with a half-hour workout. Even after that, it's a good idea to add *slowly* to the time and intensity of your activity. Eventually, you'll be able to take that five-mile run with no problem—and without injury!

THE I-DON'T-HAVE-TIME-TO-STRETCH SYNDROME

It only takes five or ten minutes, but it's amazing how many people claim they can't spare the time. The truth is, if you don't stretch, you'll end up feeling extremely sore and you'll have a much greater chance of hurting a muscle or tearing a tendon or ligament (those are what hold muscles and bones together). No matter what the excuse, it's worth the extra five or ten minutes to prevent injury.

THE BUT-I-LIKED-THE-COLOR-AND-THEY-WERE-ON-SALE SYNDROME

We'll go into this more in Chapter Seven, but, for the moment, remember that while style matters, comfort matters *more*. Especially when it comes to exercise *shoes*. If your shoes are too short or too narrow, too big or too wide, you're not only going to have foot trouble, you're going to have trouble all the way up your legs. Shoes are the most important piece of athletic clothing, so buy them in a good store where knowledgeable salespeople will measure you and make sure you get the right fit. Also, be certain that your exercise clothes aren't too tight, and don't have extraneous pieces (like bows, scarves, sharp decorations, etc.) which could get in your way or hurt you when you're working out.

THE WHY-SHOULD-I-DRINK-WATER-IF-I-DON'T-FEEL-THIRSTY? SYNDROME

As you probably remember from science class, your body is about sixty-five percent water. Water is something you need a lot of; in fact, you almost can't get too much of it. However, like most people, you probably don't get enough of it. You should drink at least four eight-ounce glasses of water a day, plus four glasses of another liquid, like tea, juice or diet soda—excluding milk, which you should think of as a food, not a beverage. Try to drink as many as six glasses of water a day. Water flushes the fats and wastes out of your body, and keeps things running smoothly.

In addition, water is essential to the exerciser.

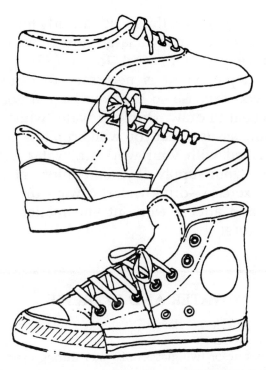

A pair of sneakers is probably the most important piece of exercise equipment you'll ever own, so choose carefully.

When you work out you lose a lot of water—the very thing that keeps you going! It is absolutely crucial to drink water before you exercise—and not just when it's hot. Everyone perspires during exercise, and even if you don't perspire heavily, you still lose a lot of water that way. If you perspire a lot, you can lose so much water that you become dehydrated—in other words, your body can lose all the water it needs to function. The frightening results include dizziness, bad headaches and even fainting.

59

By the time you're thirsty, it's already too late. You have to give your body a large store of water before you can expect it to work for you. To prevent a serious depletion, it is necessary to drink water before you exercise so that you have a good store from which to draw. Drinking water while you are exercising assures that you won't run low. After you are finished with your workout, water helps you replenish your supply. If you are thirsty at any time during exercise—drink water! Always drink before, during and after a workout—no matter what the temperature!

WATER AND EXERCISE

Drink one large glass of water ten to twenty minutes before exercise.

Drink one or two glasses of water during every half an hour that you exercise.

Drink several glasses of water when you are through.

STOP AT THE WORD OUCH

Although it isn't uncommon to get hurt when you exercise or participate in sports, it need not be an everyday occurrence. First of all, there are ways of preventing injury (some of which we've discussed above). Secondly, there are ways of treating injuries so they heal quickly.

But first, we need to get a couple of things straight about pain. There's an expression—No Pain, No

Gain—that a lot of people in sports, especially hard-core jocks, like to quote. What they mean is that if working out doesn't hurt you, you aren't really working out. So you aren't really getting any benefit. Sounds good, doesn't it? Well, it's not. In fact, it's dumb. If you're smart and careful, you don't have to get hurt or feel pain when you exercise.

Pain is your body's way of telling you that you're doing something *wrong*, and that you should stop. There's an old joke: A man goes to a doctor and says, "Doctor, doctor, it hurts when I do this!" And the doctor says, "So, stop doing that!" Makes sense, doesn't it?

The tricky part of getting in shape is knowing the difference between discomfort and pain. Sure, when you start exercising for the first time you're bound to feel some aches. You'll be using muscles you never knew you had, and you'll be flexing and stretching parts of you that never flexed or stretched before. These muscles are going to make themselves felt!

Only *you* can decide whether what you're feeling is discomfort or pain. When it *is* pain, you must stop whatever you're doing and take care of the injury—immediately! This includes resting up until you feel better. Unfortunately, once most people get into a routine of exercise, they don't want to stop. They keep using injured muscles, and the injury only gets worse! Then they really have to stop, and for a longer period of time.

Don't try to be a super jock and keep going when you're really hurt.

Watch out for these warning signs:

- ✪ *Something hurts you for more than a couple of days.*
- ✪ *The pain bothers you all day long.*
- ✪ *The pain keeps you from sleeping at night.*
- ✪ *The pain affects the way you walk or move your arms or body.*
- ✪ *There is redness or swelling accompanied by pain that lasts for more than a day or two.*

THE FIRST THING TO DO IS . . .

You guessed it—tell Mom or Dad! Whenever you feel any kind of pain, your first step ought to be to mention it to one of your parents. Your mom or dad may know exactly what to do about it (parents are like that!) or may want to call your doctor.

RICE

No, you don't have to eat rice. This is an acronym (a word made up of the first letters of several words) that is trusted by athletes. It stands for **Rest, Ice, Compression** and **Elevation.** These are the four steps you should take in treating your injury. Let's explore each one.

Rest: At the risk of disrupting your schedule, you should stay off the injury until it feels better. This is one of the reasons it's helpful to have a couple of activities that you alternate. For example, if you've hurt an arm muscle playing tennis, you might find that you can bicycle without further injury to that muscle. Go slowly and see how it feels: If it increases your discomfort at all, stop!

Ice: Ice always helps and never hurts. Heat, on the other hand, can hurt an injury, so avoid heating pads. Applying an ice pack to an injured area is easy, and it does wonders. It relieves pain, reduces swelling and lessens any bleeding. (Note: If you have excessive bleeding that doesn't seem to be stopping, it's a good idea to call your doctor.)

Never apply ice directly to your skin. Get a cold compress or place crushed ice cubes in a plastic bag and wrap a thin towel around it. Then apply it to the injury.

Compression: Wrapping up an injured limb also helps. Bind the area firmly, but not so tightly that you cut off the blood supply (you'll know you've done this if the wrapped area starts to feel numb). Also, alternate wrapping and unwrapping: Keep the injury wrapped for about half an hour, then leave it unwrapped for half an hour, wrap it again, and repeat the cycle a few times. This helps pump the blood back toward the heart, which reduces swelling and also lessens the chances of scar tissue forming.

Elevation: Keep the injured part raised higher than your heart, even while you sleep, if possible. This reduces any pressure and helps stop bleeding. This is especially good for leg and foot injuries.

WHEN TO GET PROFESSIONAL HELP

If the pain, swelling or redness lasts for more than a couple of days, even after you've dutifully tried RICE, you should think about seeing a doctor. Talk it over with your mother or father first, and let them judge.

You might also talk to some other professionals—like your gym teacher, one of the athletic coaches at school or your aerobics class instructor. Describe how you think you got the injury, what it feels like, and how you've treated it so far. Listen to their advice. But, at the risk of repeating ourselves, we'll say it one more time: If it keeps on hurting, listen to your body and your mom or dad, and go see a doctor!

☆☆   PAINLESS QUIZ   ☆☆

1. *Before exercising you:*
   a. Drink a big glass of milk for strong bones.
   b. Drink a big glass of water.
   c. Don't drink anything; you don't want to get cramps.
2. *When stretching you:*
   a. Stretch everything.
   b. Stretch your legs only if you're running.
   c. So who stretches, anyway?
3. *When shopping for exercise clothes, your biggest concern is:*
   a. How it looks.
   b. What it costs.
   c. How comfortable and practical it is.
4. *If you've swum 20 laps one week, the next week you should:*
   a. Swim 100 laps—it's worth a try.
   b. Swim 30 laps—it's not that much more.
   c. Swim 22 laps—that's ten percent.

5. *When something hurts, you know:*
   a. You're making progress.
   b. You're doing something wrong, so you try something else instead.
   c. You're doing something wrong, and you stop immediately.
6. *If the pain goes on all night, you:*
   a. Use the extra time to study.
   b. Call a doctor.
   c. Try a different exercise and hope it goes away.
7. *RICE is:*
   a. A macrobiotic eating plan.
   b. The solution to all your exercise injury problems.
   c. An acronym that stands for a good way of dealing with injuries.

Add up the points for your score:

1) a. 1	b. 2	c. 0
2) a. 2	b. 1	c. 0
3) a. 0	b. 1	c. 2
4) a. 0	b. 1	c. 2
5) a. 0	b. 1	c. 2
6) a. 0	b. 2	c. 1
7) a. 0	b. 1	c. 2

If you scored 12–14: You exercise animal, you. You're doing great.

If you scored 5–11: Not bad, but not good enough. Review the answers you got wrong, and then you'll truly be exercising safely.

If you scored 0–4: Um, well, maybe you should read this chapter again.

☆☆☆

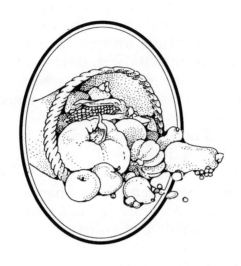

Food for Fitness

You are what you eat. Do you want to be a spongy, puffy doughnut, or a lean stalk of asparagus? Asparagus, right? Us, too.

It's a simple little phrase—you are what you eat—but it's also the absolute truth. What you eat will show in your weight, your muscle tone and your hair, skin and teeth. What you eat and drink will also affect your performance in the sports and activities in which you engage. That's why you've probably heard about things like runners' diets, and long-distance cyclists who pack fruit to eat along the way. In turn, exercise will affect your diet. People who exercise are rewarded by being able to eat more, too! Exercise speeds up their metabolism and burns off calories.

The good news is that eating right is very simple and can be delicious, too. Let's look at the basics of nutrition so you can understand why some foods are better for you than others. Then we'll talk a little about what you should eat and about the relationship between food and exercise.

ENERGIZE YOURSELF

Food is fuel to run your body. (We know it's hard to think of a pepperoni pizza this way, but it's true.) When you digest food, it's broken down, or metabolized, into chemical elements your body can use. All foods are made up of three basic elements or nutrients: *carbohydrates*, *proteins* and *fats*. Each of these is an energy source, but they're found in different foods and they provide their energy in different ways.

CARBOHYDRATES

Carbohydrates (we'll call them carbs, for short) are your body's best source of energy, and they also help to metabolize protein and fat. Not all carbs are alike. In fact, there are three kinds: the good, the very good and the awful.

The good carbs are the *simple carbohydrates* that are found in fresh fruit. Simple carbohydrates are quick energy foods which are vital to exercise. When you eat a peach, an apple or a banana, it's metabolized very quickly, giving you an immediate burst of energy which you can translate into exercise.

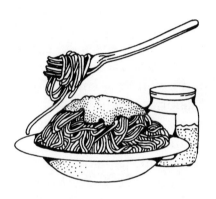

The very good carbs are *complex carbohydrates.* These are found in fresh vegetables—like broccoli, asparagus, carrots, squash, lettuce, tomatoes and potatoes—and in grain products like oats, whole wheat, brown rice, pasta (yes, pasta!) and barley. Complex carbohydrates are usually low in calories and they are metabolized more slowly, so they provide you with energy over several hours. They are good to eat during any meal prior to strenuous exercising, because they have a lasting effect. (For example, marathon runners often have pasta the night before a big race.)

The awful carbs are simple carbohydrates called *processed carbohydrates*—they include candy, ice cream and cake. There are a lot of reasons why we call these "awful." First of all, they're all made with processed sugar. That's a simple carbohydrate that is immediately taken into your blood stream and gives you a quick burst of energy. The problem is that the energy lasts only a short time, and then you suddenly feel tired. Then you need a little more sugar to sustain a high. If this sound suspiciously like an addiction, it's because that's exactly what it is.

Another reason that processed carbohydrates are in the "awful" category is that they tend to contain fat in combination with the sugar. This mixture adds up to a lot of calories. We'll talk about calories later, but you probably already know the basic fact about calories—consume too many of them and you'll find you can't fit into your jeans!

Before we go on, we'd like to set your mind at ease—we don't intend to tell you that you have to give up ice cream, cookies or candy for the rest of your life to stay fit. You just need to find the right balance for them in your total diet. We'll get to that in just a bit. First, let's finish up the basics.

PROTEIN

Another important energy source is *protein*. Actually, it serves an even more important function: Your body is primarily made up of protein. Your muscles, bones, skin, hair, nails and internal organs are all composed of protein and need it to thrive. Only protein can make the new cells that replace those cells that are worn out or damaged. Protein is found in meats, fish, poultry and dairy products such as milk, cheese and eggs. Nuts, seeds and grains also contain protein, but they're called incomplete proteins and lack the protein power of meats and dairy products. Incidentally, most foods high in protein are also pretty high in fat, which is not such a good thing!

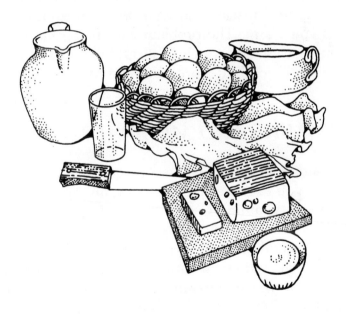

FAT

Now *fat* has a very bad reputation, which in many ways is justified. Fat contains a lot of calories. On top of that, the body burns them very slowly. Fat is found in oils, which tend to be the main ingredient in salad dressings, and they're also found in meat and in dairy products like butter and whole milk.

Still, fat isn't *all* bad, because you need some fat in your diet. Fat helps make use of some of the minerals you take into your body, and forms a cushion for your organs (like your heart and your brain), your muscles and your bones. It even helps keep you warm. The problem with fat is that most people eat far too much of it, and eventually they have too much of it stored in their bodies.

VITAMINS AND MINERALS

Vitamins and minerals are essential to a healthy diet. If you exercise, there are certain vitamins and minerals—vitamins C and E, and B-complex vitamins, as well as iron and calcium—which are particularly good for you, and you should always make sure to get adequate amounts. A good way of judging if you are getting enough of a particular vitamin or mineral is to check the U.S. recommended daily allowance for each nutrient, and to supplement your diet if you find you're falling short.

AN ATHLETE'S NUTRIENT CHART

Nutrient	What It Does	Where To Get It
Vitamin C	Helps in the formation and strengthening of bones and teeth.	Citrus fruits, raw cabbage, cantaloupe, strawberries, tomatoes and potatoes.
Vitamin E	Aids production of red blood cells, muscles and other tissues.	Vegetable oils and whole-grain breads and cereals.
B-complex vitamins	Helps skin, body's use of oxygen, protein, fat and carb metabolism and production of red blood cells.	Whole-grain breads and cereals, green leafy veggies, lean meat, eggs and all dairy products, fish, poultry, peanuts, bananas and yams.
Iron	Helps oxygen-carrying red blood cells.	Liver, shellfish, lean meat and green and yellow veggies.
Calcium	Promotes strong teeth and bones.	Milk, cheese, broccoli and spinach.

SOME OF THIS, SOME OF THAT

Finding the right balance of foods—carbs, proteins, fat and vitamins and minerals—is the key to staying healthy, trim and fit. It's also the key to maintaining a strong source of energy while you exercise. The balance is simple: Your daily diet should consist mostly of carbohydrates (more of the complex kind than the simple kind), with some protein and some fat. You can use the formula 60/15/25 to remember how much of each to eat. That means sixty percent of your calorie intake should be carbohydrates, fifteen percent should be protein and twenty-five percent (at the most) should be fat. This is broken down by calories; although it looks as if you should eat a lot of fat, you have to remember that fat has a lot of calories, which means you should actually eat very little of it!

But you don't have to be a math genius to eat right. Look at an average meal. If you had a small breast of chicken, with a baked potato with sour cream, broccoli, a whole-wheat roll with butter and then some cantaloupe for dessert, you'd end up with pretty much the 60/15/25 formula. The chicken is the fifteen percent protein, the veggies, potato and bread are complex carbs and the cantaloupe is the simple carb—which adds up to about the sixty percent of the meal. The butter and sour cream are, of course, the twenty-five percent fat. Notice that you're getting lots of vitamins, iron and calcium as well.

The meal we just described is an average, healthy meal. If you consider another kind of average meal—say, a cheeseburger, fries and soda—you get very different percentages. The fat content in this meal—between the fat used to fry the fries and burger, the fat in the burger and the fat in the cheese—is about forty percent of the total calories in the meal. The protein in the cheese and meat makes up about another forty percent. The potato is maybe ten percent for your complex carbs. The bun is really a processed carb, because it's made with white, processed flour. The soda, if it's regular, is another "awful carb"—nothing but sugar and carbonated water. That adds up to about 20/40/40: twenty percent carbs, forty percent protein and forty percent fat.

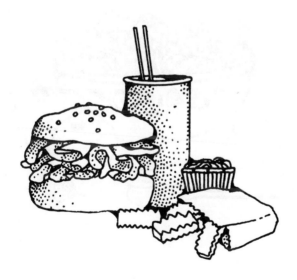

We know it's hard to avoid this kind of meal when you're out with friends or trying to get a quick lunch between classes. Besides, sometimes a burger and fries just taste good. And that's the key: Leave this kind of meal for *sometimes*. Stick with the healthy combinations for the majority of the time.

There's more to balance than just eating the right kinds of foods—although that's a big part of it. Balance is also a factor in how much you should eat and how often. It's really up to you to decide how much food you need. Eating to satisfy hunger, instead of eating when you're *not* hungry or continuing to eat when you're feeling full, is the best measure of how much you should eat.

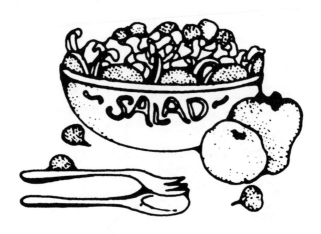

THE BEST LOW-CALORIE, NUTRITIOUS FOODS

These are some examples of good, healthy foods. This is just a starting point. From here, you should discover and add more to the list.

COMPLEX CARBS

Vegetables: broccoli, cabbage, string beans, zucchini, spinach, carrots, peas, asparagus, tomatoes, artichokes, lettuce

Breads & Cereals: whole wheat, protein bread, oatmeal, shredded wheat, bran cereals, pasta, rice

SIMPLE CARBS

Fruits: bananas, apples, oranges, grapefruit, lemons, nectarines, pineapples, plums, strawberries, peaches

PROTEIN

Poultry: white-meat chicken and turkey (remove the skin, and you remove excess fat and calories)

Other Meat: lean veal

Fish: flounder, tuna in water, sole, swordfish, bass, salmon, trout, halibut

FATS

olive oil, vegetable oils (except palm or coconut oil)

LISTEN TO YOUR STOMACH

Too many people eat because the food looks or smells good—like when you pass a bakery and are tempted by the aroma of doughnuts or the sight of the chocolate chip cookies in the window. Maybe you eat because your friend's mom offers you some pie she's just baked, or because you're at a party and the food is just there, or because you feel nervous or bored and have nothing else to do.

Although you certainly should not make yourself feel deprived and miserable, you should be careful about getting into the habit of eating when you're not hungry. First of all, if you eat when you're not hungry you're probably taking in more calories than your body needs to maintain its normal weight. And you might eventually lose your ability to tell when you really *are* hungry. Then how will you ever know when to stop?

If you want to know what's "normal," we can give you the basic guidelines: Most people get hungry about three times a day. It's usually a good idea to stick to this three-meal-a-day plan, and allow yourself some fruit in between meals if you get hungry. If, instead of eating three meals, you pick a little here and there throughout the day, you can really lose track of how much you're eating.

And remember that nature has created some foods in portions—an apple is a portion—and food companies usually put portion sizes on labels. By the way, you should get in the habit of reading food labels on packaged foods. They'll always tell you the ingredients and the suggested portion size, and they frequently include the calories and the nutritional value.

TAKE HUMAN BITES

You know how your grandparents or parents always warned you to eat slowly and chew your food thoroughly. It was not because they wanted to correct your table manners—well, maybe, sort of—but because of a rather odd scientific fact. Your stomach and your brain are about twenty minutes apart from one another. When you feel hungry, it's your stomach telling your brain that you need food. When you eat, it takes about twenty minutes for the message to travel from your stomach to your brain to signal that you've been fed. Eat slowly, even when you're ravenous, eat normal portions and wait for the message to get to your brain.

CALORIES, DIETS AND OTHER "UNFUN" THINGS

If you eat a good balance of foods (mostly complex carbs, some simple carbs, a little protein, very little fat and very few processed carbs), eat only when you're hungry, stick with three meals a day and try to avoid snacks (except for healthy snacks, like fruit), you may never have to worry about counting calories or going on a diet.

But if you do want to count calories, here are the basics: For every 3500 calories you take in *beyond what your body needs*, you could gain one pound of body fat.

You probably only need about 1500 to 2000 calories a day to maintain your normal weight. If you ate three well-balanced meals every day of the week and also had an ice cream cone each afternoon after school (the average ice cream cone is about 250 calories), cookies on Saturday (five chocolate chip cookies are about 250 calories) and a sundae on Sunday (about 500 calories), by the end of the week you'd have consumed 2,000 calories more than you need to maintain your weight. In two weeks of this kind of eating, you'd be up to 4,000 extra calories—more than enough to put on an extra pound. If you kept it up, you'd put on two pounds every month, or twenty-four pounds a year!

Exercise, as we've said, will burn calories and generally speed up your metabolism. But to burn off that sundae, you'd need to run at least five miles, play nearly two hours of tennis or do an hour of aerobics! If you feel you *have* to work out to take off the extra calories, it really takes the fun out of it.

Once you've become overweight, it's hard to lose the weight. Most girls and women must eat less than 1200 or 1000 calories a day to lose just one pound in a week (if they don't exercise). Since it's a lot easier to put on weight than it is to lose it, you're better off if you just use a little moderation in your everyday eating. Don't have the ice cream every day—have it just once a week. Instead of five cookies, eat three. Your bathing suit will thank you!

TREATS

We're only human. Go ahead and have a treat once in a while! But—there did have to be a "but," didn't there?—do it in moderation and remember that some treats are better for you than others. This means they're more nutritious and/or lower in calories. Try eating:

- ✪ *Unbuttered popcorn instead of potato chips*
- ✪ *Sorbet or frozen yogurt instead of ice cream*
- ✪ *Oatmeal cookies instead of chocolate chip cookies*
- ✪ *Angel food cake instead of brownies*
- ✪ *Fresh fruit instead of any of these!*

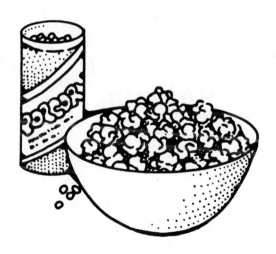

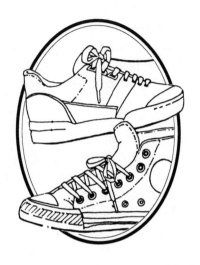

All Dressed Up . . . and Going Someplace!

*O*nce upon a time, exercise clothes meant gym clothes, and those were usually drab, baggy uniforms. Thankfully, those days are long gone! Now exercise clothes are bright, colorful and fun to wear—so much fun that people are even wearing them when they're not exercising. An added plus—

exercise clothes are now made with specific sports in mind. They allow you to move more comfortably and, in some cases, may even protect you from injury.

But there's more to exercise clothes: Wearing appropriate clothes can make you *look* the part, which, in turn, can make you *feel* more confident. If you look like a runner or a tennis player or a skier, chances are you'll feel like you really fit in and know what you're doing. Great clothes don't automatically turn you into a super athlete, of course, but they can make you feel good. In Chapter One, we talked about the relationship between feeling good and looking good, and how it goes around in a circle. Here is an extension of that rule: The more you *look* like an athlete, the more you'll *feel* like an athlete— and the more you'll *be* an athlete.

After you've selected an activity and decided to stick with it, you might want to invest in a nice outfit or two. It can be one of your rewards to yourself for keeping fit.

SMART SHOPPING

FIRST STOP—YOUR CLOSET

Sports clothes come in as many makes and styles as everyday clothes. In fact, sports clothes are so fashionable, we bet you've already got a lot of clothes in your closet that you could use for any of the activities you might want to try. Do you have sneakers, running shoes, aerobic shoes or tennis shoes? What about some cotton T-shirts? Sweats?

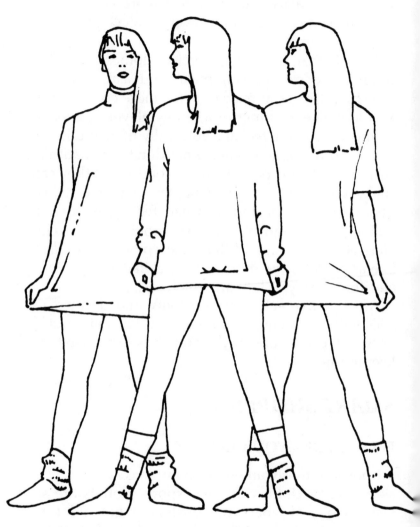

Exercise clothes are not only great for working out—they look terrific and are comfortable too!

Bike shorts? A bathing suit? We thought so. So, our first buying tip is don't buy anything until you see what you already have. You'll probably try out a couple of activities, and you don't want to invest too much of your money on clothes until you know which activities you're going to stick with.

HOT- AND COLD-WEATHER DRESSING

Hot Weather: Little, Loose and Light

In hot weather, you should wear as little as possible. Loose clothes are best, since they won't rub your skin and give you rashes. And light colors don't attract the sun (and heat) as much as dark colors do.

Cold Weather: Layered

When you go out to exercise in cold weather, there's a temptation to bundle up. But within ten minutes of starting your workout, your body temperature is going to rise to keep you warm. On the other hand, you don't want to *under*dress either.

The solution is to dress in layers, so you can take off the top layers as you get warm in the workout, then put them back on when you're cooling down at the end. And always wear a hat—otherwise you'll lose a lot of your body heat.

FIT + FASHION = THE RIGHT CHOICE

Of the two factors—fit and fashion—fit (comfort) must come first. Clothes can only be comfortable if they fit correctly, and only you can decide that. You should always try clothes on before buying them. Don't believe labels that say "one size fits all," because sometimes they don't. Don't think that something marked "medium" will fit you just because you usually take a size medium.

When trying clothes on, make sure you move around a little bit to test them out. If the outfit, or the shoe, pinches or binds or seems even a little tight or small, get the next larger size. Tight sports clothes aren't attractive—they're just uncomfortable.

Be very careful about things like seams and bindings. If the clothes have bulky seams or bindings, stay away from them. When you work out, you move a lot and you perspire. Your clothes could stick to your skin and rub. If there's a bulky seam or binding rubbing against you, you're going to end up with a rash or a blister.

FABRICS

Get in the habit of checking labels for fabric content. In general, natural fabrics like cotton and wool are good bets because they "breathe"—that is, they let air pass through the material so you don't get too hot.

In addition to the natural fabrics, there are a variety of synthetic fabrics that work really well for certain sports: Lycra tights and tops that are sold for aerobics and biking, for example. These form a kind of second skin, and "breathe" with you. A nylon jacket, on the other hand, won't breathe; it'll keep you warm by holding in your body heat. So, if you're prone to overheating, avoid nylon. In general, avoid rayon and polyester in sports clothes: They just don't breathe.

There are some new synthetics, like polypropylene, that are a little more expensive, but work almost magically. Polypropylene is a fabric that keeps you warm or cool depending on the material it's combined with—wool, cotton or nylon. Above all, it keeps you dry by drawing moisture away from your body to the outside of the fabric. This is called wicking. Usually, clothes made with these special synthetics will include a tag that explains just what they do.

PROTECTIVE GEAR

Sports clothes should not only be fashionable and comfortable, they should also keep you safe and injury-free! There are different types of protective gear needed for different sports:

Padding: Most biking shorts come with padding (terry cloth and/or moleskin) in the crotch to cushion your pubic area from the hard bicycle seat and the bumps you take as you ride. It might also be helpful for various sports, such as volleyball or roller skating, to get knee, elbow, shoulder or chest pads.

Color: Believe it or not, color is an *extremely* important safety feature. You've probably noticed that a lot of skiing, running and biking clothes come in some very loud color combinations or hot, Day-Glo colors. This is more than a fashion statement. Tests have shown that car drivers are more likely to see a runner or a biker wearing these bright colors than one dressed in a dull, single color. Iridescent white and reflective clothing—especially neon pink—are great attention-getters and are extremely good protection at night. You can even buy Velcro strips of neon colors at most athletic stores, and attach them to your exercise clothing. So be loud and colorful and safe!

Eye gear: Protective eye gear is very important in all sports and a must in some, such as racquetball. If you wear glasses, make sure they have shatterproof plastic lenses—most eyeglasses do. Even so, you'll find "grippers" useful to keep your glasses from slipping off (these are the additions that attach to the earpiece of your glasses and curl around your ears). You might want to think about contact lenses if you're going in for ball or contact sports, as they don't fall off or get broken as easily.

Headgear: When biking, helmets are of the utmost importance and *must* be worn at all times.

FOR UNDEFEATED FEET

There are many different kinds of sneakers out there, and it seems like more and more varieties are being invented every day—walking shoes, running shoes, racing shoes, tennis shoes, basketball shoes, boating shoes, bicycling shoes, warm-up shoes, aerobic shoes, cross-training shoes, etc. It seems a bit ridiculous. How are you ever supposed to know which ones you should wear?

Well, basically, try to ignore all the hype. The three main features that any athletic shoe should have are comfort, support and durability. They should be extremely comfortable, with lots of padding where it's needed and a good, thick sole. They should provide support where necessary, at the arch or at the ankle (depending on the sport). And they should last. The final requirement, durability, is fairly easy to determine—leather lasts longer than suede, and suede is sturdier than cloth (but cloth is usually a lot cheaper, so sometimes it's worth it!).

The three sports for which you should seriously consider getting "special shoes" are running, bicycling and aerobics. A good running shoe has lots of padding and gives you support all along the bottom of the shoe, especially in the arch. There are special "cleated" biking shoes you can purchase, but, in general, all you need is a good, firm sneaker with a stiff sole (you don't want your feet to "bend"). For aerobics, you should get a well-padded, supportive shoe that has a high ankle-piece and a good, strong arch support. You do quite a bit of bouncing in aerobics, so you need to be very well cushioned and supported.

For all other sports, you'll either be told exactly what type of shoe to get by your team (for example, for soccer you might need cleats, for tennis a white-soled shoe, etc.) or you can make do with any well-made sneaker you like.

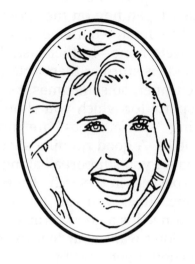

Listen Up! Your Body Is Talking

Your body is changing. Girls between the ages of ten and thirteen begin to experience pretty dramatic changes in the way they look and feel. It can be a little overwhelming at times, but basically this is a really exciting time of your life. You're becoming a woman, with a woman's body and a woman's concerns. It is the beginning of something new, so like all firsts—your first day at school, your first piano recital or your first date—you might feel a little in the dark, as if everyone else knows something you don't know. Relax. Everyone's confused, frightened and excited by these new experiences and changes. In this chapter, we want to give you a quick review of what you can expect to happen during these years and why. As you read, we want you to remember two important things:

Never be afraid to ask questions. Growing up and going through puberty are complicated processes. The changes you experience can be scary, especially if you don't know what to expect. And even after you read this chapter or other books on the subject, you'll probably still have questions. Never, never be embarrassed or afraid to ask those questions. Ask your parents or your doctor, the school nurse or your teacher. Ask an older sister or a friend, whomever you trust and believe has the right information. They may not always know the answers, but they can probably tell you where to go to get them. The important thing is to ask if you have a question, because it's your body and you have a right to know about it and be comfortable with it.

Everyone develops differently. That's because everyone is unique. Think about it—do you know anyone who is exactly like you? Unless you have an identical twin, you don't. Don't expect that you will develop exactly like anyone else, and don't worry when you don't. You'll develop at your own pace, as the unique person you are. You may be a late bloomer, or an early bloomer, or a steady bloomer. But we guarantee that you will bloom!

WHAT YOU CAN EXPECT

Basically, puberty is when our bodies change from being girls' bodies to being women's bodies. These changes can start as early as eight for some girls, and as late as sixteen for others. Most girls start to notice these changes around age twelve. All of the changes that you go through during puberty are brought about by *hormones*—chemicals in the blood that regulate virtually all of your bodily functions. This is true for boys as well (it's just that boys have different hormones).

We're going to review the changes more or less in the order they will occur—but remember, the sequence won't be exactly the same for everyone. You may be first among your friends to reach your full, adult height, and the last to get your period. Sooner or later, though, you're going to experience every one of these changes.

HEIGHT AND BONES

First of all, you'll experience a spurt in growth. All of your bones are part of this spurt, but they don't all grow at the same rate. As a result, you may go through stages where things seem all out of proportion—but don't worry, it will all even out in the end. Your head, hands and feet will probably grow first—they'll reach their adult proportions before you've reached your full height. If it suddenly feels like your feet are too big for your body, just remember the rest of you will catch up soon. Next come the legs and arms—that's the stage when it may seem that you're totally uncoordinated, and you can't figure out where to put those long legs that have suddenly sprouted. Again, don't worry. Your "trunk," the spine and torso, is the last major bone group to grow.

SHAPE, MUSCLE AND FAT

Your body shape will change during puberty, and become more curvy. Your hips will grow wider and more fat will be deposited around your thighs, buttocks, and stomach and, of course, in your breasts. And, even though you're getting curvier, your muscles will also be developing and getting denser. Even the shape of your face will change, generally lengthening and becoming fuller. If you exercise during this time, you can have a lot of control over the final shape of your body. Your present efforts to become shapely and muscular will improve your body for the rest of your life.

HAIR AND SKIN, OIL AND PERSPIRATION

You'll begin to grow a lot more hair—on your arms and legs, under your arms and in your pubic area—and the hair may be darker, denser and curlier. Your skin and the hair on your head will become oilier. That increased oil will begin to bring on some mild skin problems in almost all girls—pimples, blackheads and whiteheads just seem to be part of growing up. And you'll begin to perspire more, especially under your arms, and the perspiration will begin to have an adult odor.

SECONDARY SEX CHARACTERISTICS

That's the way they always refer to them in books. Mostly what they are referring to is pubic hair and breasts. Most girls begin to grow pubic hair first; this is followed by breast development. But for other girls it's the reverse. Both processes, though, will take anywhere from a month to two years from the time you begin to notice the changes until the time they're complete.

MENSTRUATION

Your period is actually the last and most noticeable stage of an important and complicated process that goes on inside your body. Once a month (or about every twenty-eight days), your pituitary gland (a little gland near your brain) sends a signal to your ovaries to release an egg. That egg, if fertilized by a sperm, will become a fetus. Each month your body gets ready to have the egg fertilized. It does this by making a thick, cushy lining for the uterus, where the fetus would develop. That lining is soft, new tissue, nourished by blood vessels which have swelled up with blood to sustain that tissue. When the egg isn't fertilized, it can't attach itself to this new home in the uterus. A series of chemical messages tell your body that its preparation for a fetus was unnecessary. Then the swollen blood vessels begin to shrink, and the lining begins to fall away from the uterus. The blood vessels of the lining gradually open, and tiny drops of blood are released. And that's your period.

The bleeding usually goes on for about five days (although for some girls it's three days, and for others it's seven). Then your period stops, and the cycle begins again in about two weeks, with another ovum, or egg, being released, and the uterine lining developing and then shedding.

MONTHLY MATTERS

It's a good idea to keep a record of your period. Being very irregular can be a sign of a medical problem, so your doctor will always ask whether you're regular or not. But remember, most girls don't become "regular"—in other words, get their periods at regularly spaced intervals—for at least two years. Another reason for keeping track is to reduce the element of surprise. If you know more or less when your period is due, you can be prepared with pads or tampons.

PMS AND OTHER SYMPTOMS

Prior to and during your period, you might experience some new physical and emotional sensations. PMS (or premenstrual syndrome) is the name given to these sensations. Some girls have only a few symptoms and very little discomfort, but others may have a lot. Some girls experience symptoms once their period has begun, and others experience them in the days before. This is another reason to keep track of your period—if you notice that you get the same symptoms month after month, you'll learn what to expect and what to do about it.

The symptoms associated with menstruation and premenstrual syndrome vary widely—in fact, most are exact opposites. And, though many are negative, some are very positive. Here is a list of the most common symptoms; remember, you may experience some of these or none:

- *fatigue or extra energy*
- *bloating or water retention, often resulting in a temporary weight gain*
- *increased appetite, craving for sweets*
- *breakouts or especially clear skin*
- *headaches, lower back and leg aches or stomach cramps*
- *constipation or diarrhea*
- *feelings of depression or well-being*
- *inability to concentrate or heightened concentration and creativity*

No one knows yet exactly why these symptoms occur, but they are now certain that menstrual and premenstrual symptoms are chemically based—and very real. If you suffer severe negative symptoms—such as fatigue, cramps or the inability to concentrate—talk to your mother or your doctor about it. If the symptoms are mild, there are a variety of remedies you can try, including changes in diet and, yes, exercise! On the other hand, your skin may clear up during this time and you may feel particularly happy and energized.

Incidentally, your period and the symptoms you experience may change from month to month. Some months you may experience a very light flow of blood or a few symptoms, and other months may bring a heavy flow or a lot of bothersome symptoms.

MENSTRUATION AND EXERCISE

There was a time when women hardly moved at all when they had their periods. Those were the days when it was referred to as "the curse"—as if it were a punishment that women had to suffer through!

Of course, in those days, women were generally less active. And the fact is that before tampons, swimming and other strenuous sports could be a little tricky! Fortunately, today we have better attitudes about menstruation and better ways of dealing with the flow. We now know that exercise actually tends to *reduce* the symptoms of PMS and can even minimize cramps. Doctors aren't sure why that is, but they suspect it may be those endorphins we talked about earlier. In any case, exercise won't make your period flow more heavily—or make your cramps worse. It will probably make you feel a lot better. So don't let cramps be an excuse to miss gym class!

One of these lies, though, has some truth in it. Some girls who exercise very strenuously—and we mean *very* strenuously, like professional ballet dancers who work out several hours a day, or marathon runners who log thirty or forty miles a week—might begin to miss their periods. This is called amenorrhea (pronounced ay-men-oh-ree-uh). Doctors aren't sure why it happens. It's been found that once girls cut back on exercise, their periods almost always return. Since most of you won't be taking up such strenuous programs, it's unlikely that this will happen to you; but, if you *do* stop menstruating, you should talk to your doctor about it and maybe he or she can suggest ways to restructure your exercise plan.

☆☆ WHAT'S "NORMAL" IN ☆☆ DEVELOPMENT QUIZ

1. *The proportions you have at age twelve are the ones you'll keep for the rest of your life.*
   True or False
2. *If your breasts don't start to develop early, you probably will be small-breasted.*
   True or False

3. *Some girls don't get their first period until they're fifteen or sixteen.*
   True or False
4. *Not everyone gets terrible cramps with their first period.*
   True or False
5. *The symptoms you get with your first period are the same ones you'll always have.*
   True or False
6. *Before or during their periods, all girls get depressed, or experience some other PMS symptom.*
   True or False

And the answers:

1. **False.** Your bones grow at different rates, so your proportions will be changing all through your teen years.

2. **False.** Some girls begin to develop late, but then grow very quickly.

3. **True.** And that's still within the range considered "normal."

4. **True.** Cramps are a very common symptom, but even so, not everyone gets bad cramps. Some girls have mild cramps, and some have none at all.

5. **False.** Symptoms change from month to month and from year to year. Even the flow and the length of time you bleed changes from time to time.

6. **False.** Depression can be a PMS symptom, but so is an increased feeling of well-being, in which case it's not so much a symptom as it is a benefit.

The point is there are no firm rules here. You might experience a few "symptoms" or you might experience none at all. You might even reap some benefits!

☆☆☆

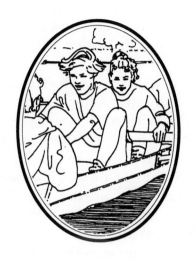

Ready, Set, Go!

*G*etting started. You guessed it—this is the hardest part. Until you actually begin exercising, you can't feel the benefits we've been talking about—so right now all you may see is the effort involved. Once you do start, though, it's easy to keep going because by then you'll know that exercise makes you feel great!

You must be convinced by now that you ought to begin, or you wouldn't still be reading. But we also know that there can be an enormous distance between knowing you should do something, and turning it into an action—that is, getting your feet moving.

One of the toughest problems facing beginners is the basic law of inertia: *A body at rest tends to remain at rest.* Why? Well, your science teacher would probably give you a different answer, but we think it's because it's easier. It's simpler for most of us to sit and do nothing, or to watch others do things, than to get ourselves moving. Just consider how much easier it is to watch a basketball game than to try to join the team and play!

Of course, there are some people who just automatically **move**. It's their nature. There's another law in physics that applies to them: *A body in motion tends to remain in motion.* Those of you who fit into this category can skip this next section, because now we're going to talk about what keeps the rest of us at rest—EXCUSES!

EXCUSES, EXCUSES!

You may find it surprising that even once you're revved up about the idea of fitness, negative thoughts keep creeping into your head, telling you why you can't, or shouldn't, begin a fitness program. You keep thinking there are more important things to do—like washing your hair or waiting for that cute guy to call or watching that soap opera— anything but exercise! Or you may try to convince yourself that exercise is not right for you. After all, you didn't sleep well last night, and you might break a nail playing tennis or make a fool of yourself in front of the team.

The good news is that you don't need to take those negative thoughts seriously. We all get them; and we all get pretty much the same ones. Now let's go through them one by one, and get rid of them once and for all!

EXCUSE #1: "BUT I'M NOT ATHLETIC!"

Everybody has *some* natural athletic ability. In order to get into shape and stay fit, you just need to find the exercise or sport that comes the most naturally to you. And, like most things, if you work at it, you will improve. Think about the things you've learned in the last few years and at which you have excelled. Things like fixing your hair, doing your homework or riding a bike. They were all hard at first, but then you practiced them and now they're second nature to you. You may not have been born a great athlete, but you can become a pretty good one if you practice.

"I'm not athletic" may really be an excuse for excuse #2.

EXCUSE #2: "BUT I'LL BE EMBARRASSED IF I DON'T DO IT RIGHT!"

Let's be honest: You may *not* do it "right" at first—it takes a little bit of time to learn anything. But you've got to remember that everyone was a beginner once, even sports giants! Anyone who is an athlete will understand. If they see that you're doing something wrong, they won't ridicule you—they'll try to teach you how to do it right. Once you get good at an exercise or sport, you'll find that you have more confidence, smoother coordination and better feelings about yourself. Embarrassment about your body and your ability will be a thing of the past. As long as you take yourself seriously, other people will, too.

EXCUSE #3: "BUT I'M TOO TIRED!"

You probably are tired—growing up takes a lot of energy, and if you don't give your body some help by keeping it in shape you will be tired. But, as you know, exercise will actually make you less fatigued! Ask yourself when you felt more tired: the last time you went to a dance, or when you sat around all day watching TV? Often, when you're bored, you feel tired. The real problem is that the less you do, the more bored and tired you get, and the less you feel like doing anything. The only way to break this cycle is to *exercise*. Once you get moving, you're sure to have more energy and more enthusiasm.

EXCUSE #4: "BUT I DON'T HAVE TIME!"

Time can be a very real problem. Most people have lots of things they want to do and very little time to do them. And so it is necessary to learn to manage your time to make room for all the things that you really want to do.

A good way to start is to make a list of all the things you do in a typical day. Some of them, like going to school, can't be changed; but you'll find that quite a few can. Check off those things that can be shifted, shortened or moved around to make time for other activities. Notice that you probably haven't filled up twenty-four hours worth of time—even if you include sleeping. Now look at your schedule and decide where you can sneak in a half an hour for exercise. For example: How much time do you spend watching television? Or on the phone with friends? Or trying to decide what you'll wear to school the next day? Or just sitting around, figuring out what to do next?

Can you skim half an hour off any of these things? Or squeeze in some time in between? Remember that an exercise program really only requires half an hour to an hour three days a week.

EXCUSE #5: "BUT IF I EXERCISE, I'LL GET THOSE GREAT BIG, BULGING MUSCLES!"

The only women who will develop bulging muscles from exercise are those who intentionally work at body building by lifting weights—and they have to work *very* hard to accomplish it. Women's muscles simply don't bulge the way men's do.

EXCUSE #6: "BUT I'LL SWEAT, AND GIRLS SHOULDN'T SWEAT!"

This one comes from the same time period when it was said women shouldn't go out in public when they were menstruating. Those were also the days when it was said that women shouldn't work or vote. So if you don't believe any of those whoppers, then you have to believe that it's okay for girls to work out, exercise and play sports—and sweat. We're no longer in the dark ages. We believe that both girls and guys are entitled to good, clean, athletic sweat when working out and keeping fit!

THE DON'Ts

Most excuses are just thoughts that will only defeat you if you let them. Once you've actually started exercising, they'll probably fade away. But there are some real pitfalls to watch out for. As in every new experience, you'll find out that there are things you shouldn't do. It's impossible to predict everything that might come up, but below are some of the common predicaments:

DON'T OVERREACH

You should begin your fitness program with something you can handle, and then gradually work your way up to more ambitious activities. If you've never exercised before and you start out with something that requires a lot of skill, like tennis, or stamina, like an hour-long aerobics class, you may find that your skill or stamina level just isn't up to snuff. Then you may get discouraged and completely give up.

In Chapter Two, we gave you a guide to assess your natural aptitudes, likes and dislikes. Using that guide, pick some activities that won't be beyond your reach. For example, if you're interested in running, you might start with walking. If you'd like to try an aerobics class, start with low-impact aerobics or a calisthenics class. If you're interested in tennis, borrow a racket from a friend and play a few friendly games before you invest in a racket and tennis club membership. Then, once you're comfortable and confident, you can be as ambitious as you like!

DON'T OVERDO

Sometimes people get carried away by enthusiasm. They feel so good when they begin exercising that they don't want to stop, and they end up overdoing it. They run four miles instead of two, take two aerobics classes in a row or play tennis until they drop. .

The upshot, unfortunately, is that they wake up the next day in pain, with enough aches and blisters to put them off exercising forever. In order to avoid this, you should follow the guidelines we've given for slowly building up your exercise program (always ten percent at a time!). In time, you'll increase your stamina and strength and be able to do whatever you want.

DON'T OVERSPEND

Although it's true that you have to give yourself some time to practice and "get good" at any activity, it's also true that you might need to experiment with several activities before you decide which one you want to pursue seriously. And until you've really made up your mind, it's pointless to spend lots of money on equipment and clothes that you may never use again.

Don't go out and buy new skis or expensive aerobic shoes until you're fairly certain that's the activity you want to pursue. Otherwise, if you want to change sports, you might not have the money for the right gear.

THE DO'S

Now let's talk about some of those things that will give you a great start:

DO COMMIT YOURSELF TO TRYING

You really need to promise yourself that you'll give exercise an honest try. One good idea is to write down your goals and plans in pursuing an exercise program. This will help focus your reasons, and can serve as a reminder if your enthusiasm flags.

Start by writing down why you want to get fit. For example:

I'm going to try exercise because:

- ✪ *I want to lose weight.*
- ✪ *I want to get stronger.*
- ✪ *I want to build up my _____.*
- ✪ *I want to meet new friends.*
- ✪ *I want to learn how to _____(play tennis, ride a bike, etc.).*
- ✪ *I want to be generally healthier.*
- ✪ *I want to _____.*

Next, write down what you are willing to do to reach that goal. Something like: "I'm going to devote at least half an hour, three times a week for the next three months, to trying out various exercises and sports until I find one that's right for me. Once I do, I'm going to devote at least one and a half hours a week to that activity."

DO KEEP A JOURNAL OF YOUR PROGRESS

Write down every activity you try and what you experience. Just little notes, like: "June 1: Ran a mile and a half without feeling winded. June 3: Took first tennis lesson, learned how to hold the racket." When you look back over your journal, you'll be amazed how quickly you've moved forward, and this will serve to inspire you to continue and achieve even more.

DO MAKE IT SOCIAL

It's always smart to exercise with another person who's also interested in beginning a fitness program. There are many reasons for this. For one,

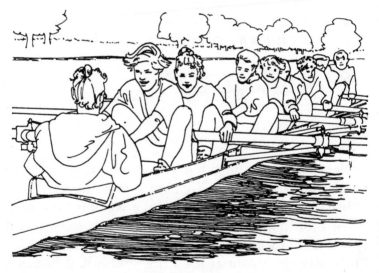

Joining a team is great for your body, and it can do wonders for your social life as well.

almost everything's more fun if you do it with a friend; for another, you and your friend can inspire one another to keep going. Hopefully, you will be able to find someone who is at about your current level of fitness, strength and ability, but if not, the two of you should simply work out at levels that are appropriate to each of you, and eventually you'll probably even out.

In addition to finding a buddy, you might want to find an exercise group or a team. For example, look around your town for the local biking or running club. Join school teams for sports that interest you. Take a class or join a gym. All the benefits of having a friend to exercise with are multiplied by having many exercise buddies!

DO EXPLORE DIFFERENT OPTIONS

Find an activity that you really enjoy, and don't give up until you do. Even if you find you like one thing, don't let that stop you from trying another. And another. You never know what you'll like, or what you may be good at, until you try it.

DO REWARD YOURSELF

After a while, you'll find that you like certain activities, and that you're making progress. Reward yourself with a new exercise outfit, or a new piece of equipment. Or give yourself a reward that isn't connected with the exercise, like buying yourself flowers or a new poster for your room. You deserve it! Remember, giving yourself things that make you look and feel better will give you more self-confidence and that, in turn, will enable you to do things that will improve you—inside and out!

DO HAVE FUN

We've said it a trillion times, but it's worth saying it again: The best reason of all to pursue an exercise program is because you enjoy it. If it makes you happy, then all the other benefits are like icing on the cake. So even though we're asking you to make a commitment and take it seriously, we don't want it to be a chore. One thing we know for sure is that if you don't enjoy the activity you pick, you won't stay with it. And if you're enjoying it, there's nothing at all to stop you!

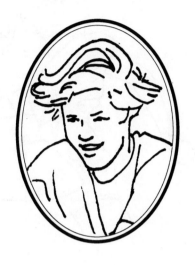

Balance and Perfection

You know now that a "great body" isn't one that someone else defines and you work to develop. You already have a great body—you just have to make it happen by achieving a balance. We know it sounds too simple, but it's true. Besides, it isn't actually all that simple. In fact, it's easier to get *off* balance. All you have to do is eat too much, or too

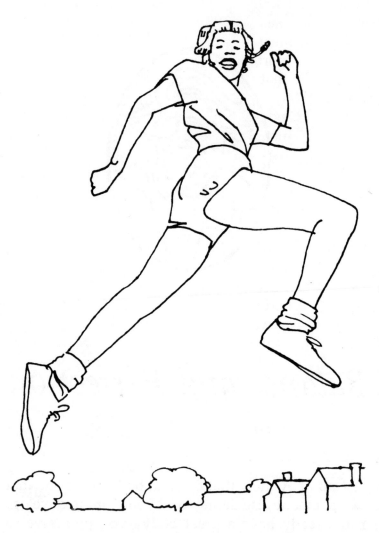

Perfection means being the best you can be!!

little, or too many of the wrong foods, or over- or under-exercise. Creating a balance for your body really just means doing everything in moderation. The tricky part is knowing how to achieve this goal. Well, that's one reason we gave you exercise schedules.

Those schedules are designed to give you an idea of what's just right. And if you remember the "magic threes"—exercise a minimum of thirty minutes three times a week, and eat three meals a day with nothing (or healthy snacks) in between—you won't have to worry about too little. As for too much: If you're exercising, that will control your appetite and your metabolism and you will probably naturally eat exactly the right amount. And heavy exercise can become bad for you only if you don't allow your body to get used to it by slowly working up to it. Anyway, other activities like school and homework, dances and dates, movies and household chores will keep you from exercising twelve hours a day!

MAKING PROGRESS

The only way you can make progress—at anything—is to set goals for yourself. We talked about setting goals in Chapter Nine. Remember what your goals were when you began reading, and think some more about them now that you've finished. Write them down in an exercise journal.

Again, you'll want to compare your actual progress with your goals once a week or so. Once again, remember, you're after progress, not perfection. If you don't match your goals perfectly, it's okay, as long as you keep trying and making progress.

A FINAL WORD ABOUT "PERFECTION"

Some of you may find yourselves making tremendous progress in one or more of the exercises or sports you choose. When that happens, when you begin to get very good at something, you'll generally want to keep at it, getting more and more "perfect" at it, and more and more serious.

Well, that's just terrific and we hope that some of you become great athletes—maybe even world-famous ones! But remember, even if you don't, you're still a winner. Being fit and thinking well of yourself are two of the most terrific things that could happen to you. So, keep exercising, have fun and remember that no matter what you do, you have the potential to be a winner.